Energize your life

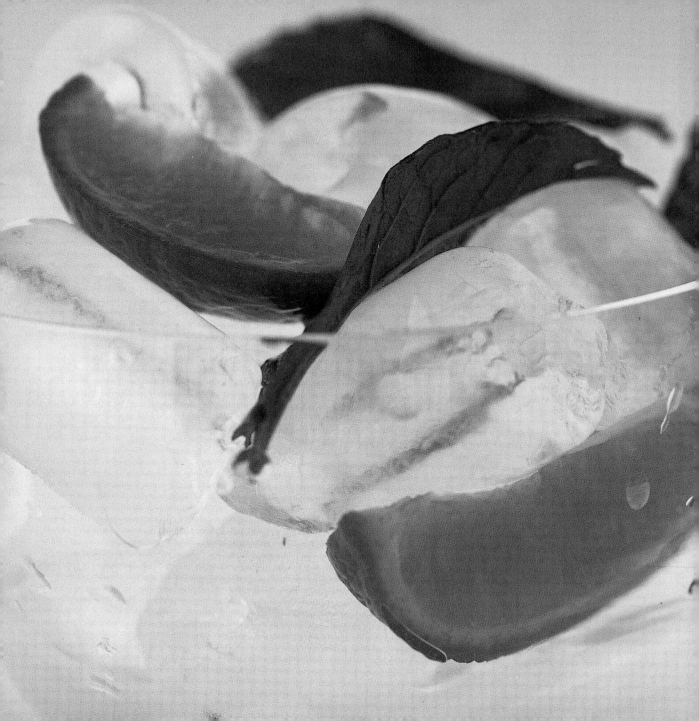

Energize
your life

Nic Rowley and Kirsten Hartvig
Emma Mitchell
Alistair Livingstone

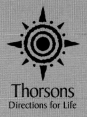

Thorsons
Directions for Life

Energize Your Life

Thorsons
An imprint of HarperCollins*Publishers*
77–85 Fulham Palace Road
Hammersmith, London, England W6 8JB

Published in the United States by Thorsons in 2002

Conceived, created, and designed by Duncan Baird Publishers.

Material from this book was first published in the USA in 2000 by
Celestial Arts in two separate volumes from the *Naturally ...* series:
Energy Exercises and *Energy Foods*.

Library of Congress Cataloging-in-Publication Data is available.

ISBN: 0-00-764061-7

10 9 8 7 6 5 4 3 2 1

Typeset in Rotis Sans Serif and Univers
Color reproduction by Colourscan, Singapore
Printed by Imago, Singapore

Publisher's note
None of the information in *Energize Your Life* is meant as a substitute for
professional medical advice. If you are in any doubt as to the suitability of
any of the exercises, therapeutic methods, or recipes given in this book,
consult your doctor. The publishers, the authors, and the photographers
cannot accept responsibility for any injuries or damage incurred as a result
of following the exercises or recipes in this book, or using any of the
therapeutic methods described or mentioned here.

"Everything rests in *prana* energy, as the spokes rest in the hub of a wheel." PRASHNA UPANISHAD

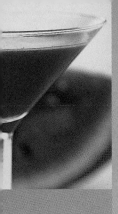

Contents

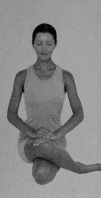

Introduction

Most cultures and traditions recognize that there is more to a human being than flesh, blood and bones. They acknowledge the existence of a vital energy which reaches beyond the physical – the essence of life. This energy is our most precious possession, and maintaining our energy flow, through diet and exercise, is the key to realizing our potential, both physically and spiritually.

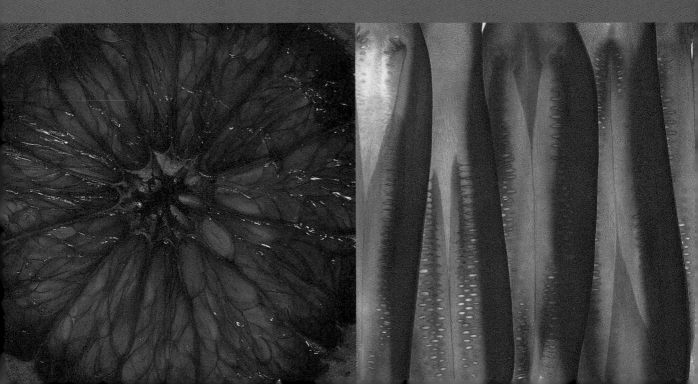

Energize Your Life is a distillation of knowledge gleaned from a range of both Eastern and Western traditions and therapies. An extensive collection of recipes allows you to put into practice the naturopathic idea that a well-nourished body is the key to a healthy life. Eastern concepts of energy are explored through a wide range of t'ai chi, qigong and yoga exercises.

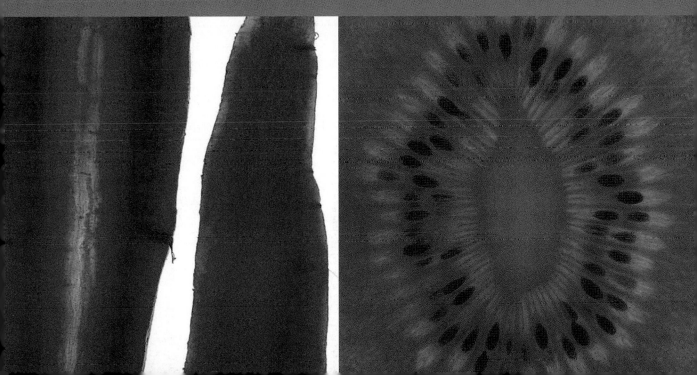

energy foods and juices

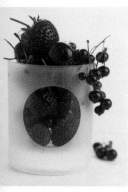

Section 1 of this book offers an overview of up-to-date nutritional knowledge blended with proven naturopathic wisdom to help you create a new and exciting way to eat. All the breakfast, lunch, dinner, snack and juice recipes put energy food principles into practice enabling you to maximize the nutritional values of everything you eat and drink.

All the recipes are quick and easy to make. To make the fruit juices, all you need is a simple squeezer or hand press. For vegetable juices, smoothies and shakes you will need an electric juicer, food processor or electric blender. Make only as much juice as you can drink straight away.

ABOUT THE RECIPE RATING SYSTEM For quick reference, many of the recipes are given a star rating (maximum five stars) to make the energy benefits of each recipe immediately apparent.

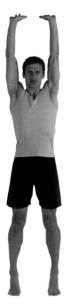

energy exercises

Section 2 of the book introduces disciplines such as t'ai chi, qigong and yoga, suggesting exercises, postures and movements to stimulate and encourage energy flow. It also features exercises based on the Western technique of kinesiology and on the therapeutic qualities of Egyptian dance. These traditions and techniques are increasingly recognized as ways to improve the appearance of the body, stay fit and prevent or treat long-term health problems.

You can do all of the exercises found in this book by yourself throughout the day, at home or at work, without the guidance of an instructor. The postures, breathing practices and relaxation techniques will help you to still your mind, revitalize your body and restore your energy levels. Many practices are modified for beginners, so that you can perform them easily and safely. Start incorporating energy exercises into your life today and feel the benefits for yourself.

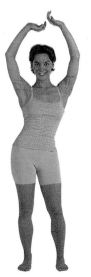

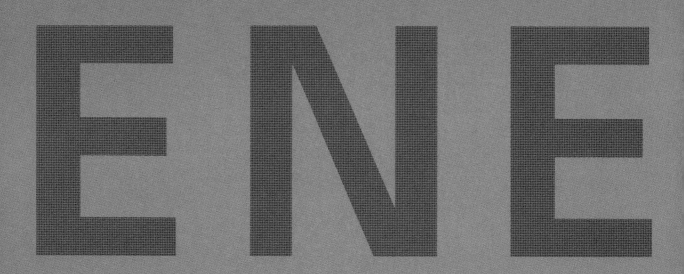

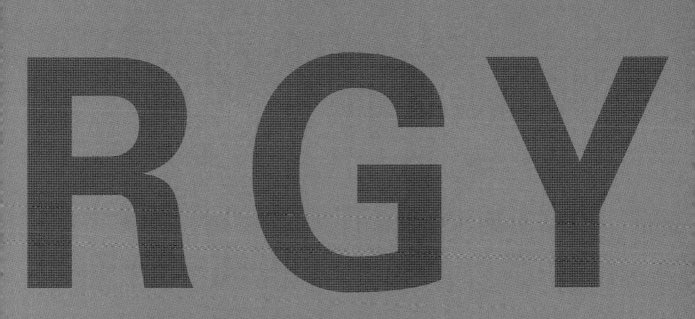

RGY
ID JUICES

section one

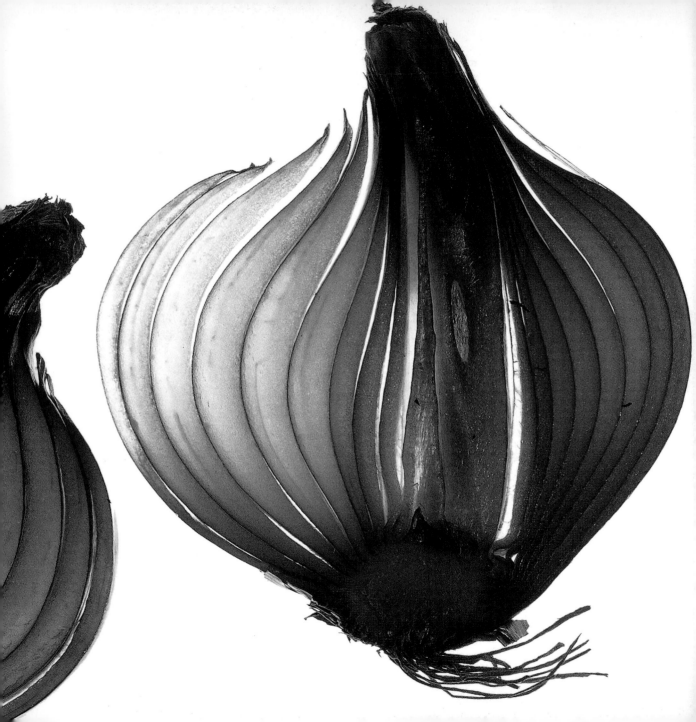

chapter one

The healthy way

If we want our bodies to be fit, and to function at peak performance level, the best long-term investment we can make is to eat and drink healthily.

By adopting a mainly plant-centered diet including fresh fruit, raw vegetables and pulses and whole grains, supplemented by plenty of fresh juices and plain water, we can provide ourselves with all the basic nutrients we need to increase our energy levels and live life to the full. Furthermore, healthy eating and drinking can stimulate our in-built capacity to heal ourselves.

Natural health awareness

In a world of rich diversity there is one thing on which scientists, scholars and sages all agree – life is the movement of energy. From first heartbeat to last breath, our bodies are constantly transforming food-energy into warmth, movement, thought, emotion and activity. By eating in tune with nature and tapping into the vitality of fresh, organic ingredients, we can move closer to the sources of life-energy – the sun and the soil – and so enhance our health and wellbeing. Here are five natural nutritional principles to help you transform your diet into one based on energy foods.

Eat fresh
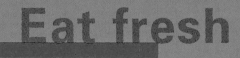

Too much refined and processed food robs the body of vital nutrients and increases our intake of fat, sugar and additives.

Eat organic
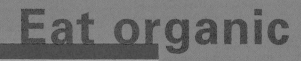

Food that is free from chemical residues and genetic manipulation improves our health and that of the planet.

Eat raw

Eating fresh fruit and raw salad each day increases our fiber and reduces our salt intake, helps to optimize our absorption of protein and ensures a rich supply of cancer-busting phytochemicals (health-enhancing substances found only in plant foods).

Eat plants

Invest in your long-term health by including more plant-based food in your diet. Try to eat more vegetables and less meat. Replace cow's milk by soy, rice, oat or almond milk, and replace butter with unhydrogenated plant spreads, free from trans-fatty acids. Use polyunsaturated plant oils (such as safflower or sunflower oil) in cooking and salad dressings.

Eat smart

Eat when you are hungry, stop when you are satisfied. Chew your food well and try not to eat when you are angry, frustrated, stressed or in a hurry. Cut down on refined sugar – use honey, and maple and fruit syrups in place of sugar whenever you can. Also decrease your intake of stimulants – beverages containing caffeine give you short-term energy at the expense of long-term vitality.

Body power

As societies have become more urbanized and developed, so the number of people suffering from the effects of heart disease, strokes and cancer has increased. At the root of these changing health patterns is the move away from a diet based on grains, fruits and vegetables to one based on processed foods, fat, sugar and animal produce.

The scientific evidence is clear: if we want to have healthy bodies, we should change our food focus and put fresh fruit, fresh vegetables, pulses and whole grains back in the center of our plates (supplemented by fresh, organically reared meat and fish according to taste). Here are some of the most important components of a healthy, energy-full diet.

Calcium

Crucial for building and maintaining healthy bones and teeth, calcium also plays an important role in the function of nerves, muscles, enzymes and hormones. Most plant foods contain calcium – spinach, watercress, parsley, dried figs, nuts, seeds, molasses, seaweed and soy are all rich suppliers. Ounce for ounce, bean curd (tofu) contains four times more calcium than whole cow's milk.

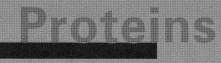

Proteins

The building blocks of the body, proteins consist of long, folded chains of amino acids. It is not widely known that plant foods contain protein and that vegetables, grains and pulses are all good sources – ounce for ounce, soy flour contains more protein than steak, and butterbeans have more than flounder.

Complex carbohydrates

Complex carbohydrates are made of sugar molecules linked together into long, branched chains. Found only in foods made from plants, they are a major source of energy in our diet and have beneficial effects on the way we absorb and use other nutrients. Foods containing complex carbohydrates, such as bread and pasta, are usually rich in vitamins, minerals and trace elements.

Antioxidants

In the process of metabolism, our body's cells produce molecules called free radicals, which can attack and harm cell membranes. Antioxidants, such as beta-carotene, vitamin C, vitamin E and selenium, neutralize these unstable chemicals, in turn protecting our cells. Fruit, vegetables, nuts, grains and cold-pressed plant oils are the main sources of antioxidants in our diet.

Essential fatty acids

Two polyunsaturated fatty acids, linoleic acid and alpha-linolenic acid, are known as essential fatty acids because they can be obtained only from the food we eat. They are necessary for normal growth of the fetus during pregnancy, and play a central role in blood-clotting and healing wounds. They also help to maintain the health of the brain and the cells of other parts of our bodies. Important sources of essential fatty acids include green leaves (such as lettuce and cabbage) and vegetable oils (for example, sunflower, safflower, wheatgerm and corn oils).

19

Brain power

energy foods for healthy minds

Energy foods benefit the brain as well as the body. They provide glucose and micronutrients, such as thiamine, riboflavin, niacin, vitamin C and iron, to maximize our mental performance and to help us cope better under pressure. They enhance the carbohydrate–protein balance in our diet to make us calmer and more alert, and improve the quality of our sleep. They also reduce our reaction to common causes of food intolerance and make us less prone to depression, headaches and general tiredness. Here are six simple ways to boost your brain power.

Kick-start vitality

Eat a good breakfast to avoid low blood sugar in the late morning, and to sharpen your memory and mental clarity. (See pp.72–5 for a selection of delicious high-energy breakfasts to launch the day.)

Snack often

Boost your vitality mid-morning and mid-afternoon with a quick-fix snack or drink (pp.92–103). These will help to keep you alert right up until the end of the day.

Eat regularly

Keep regular meal times and do not skip meals. Research shows that eating several small meals per day helps the brain to work more efficiently than having one or two big meals.

Oil the cogs

Ensure your body gets a rich supply of essential fatty acids by including salads, green, leafy vegetables and some safflower and sunflower oil in your diet. Low in saturated animal fats, energy foods are high in plant polyunsaturates, which keep our brain cells in peak condition.

Power sleep

Take a power nap after your midday meal. Brain efficiency naturally drops after lunch, and the short time it takes to recharge your batteries will more than repay itself in extra mental energy later in the day.

Pump iron

Eat more wholegrain cereals, pulses and green vegetables to boost your iron intake. Drink a glass of vitamin C-rich, fresh fruit juice each day to maximize iron absorption.

Energy burn

balancing energy input and output

Converting what we eat into energy to fuel the things we do is one of the fundamental processes of life. Here are some suggestions as to how to fine tune your energy burn for maximum health and vitality.

Sustain output

Eat more complex carbohydrates to spread out energy release from your food throughout the day, and avoid energy lows. Pasta, wholegrain bread, pulses and fresh vegetables are all good sources.

Control temperature

Keeping warm when it is cold and cool when it is hot uses a surprising amount of energy. Try to keep your body at a constant, comfortable temperature and avoid sudden changes in surroundings that make you shiver or sweat.

Stay calm

Anxiety and mental stress use up physical energy even when you are not active. Taking time to deal with these two energy drainers repays itself many times over in extra vitality gained.

Avoid stimulants

Nicotine and caffeine increase energy burn without putting new energy into the body. Avoid cigarettes, coffee, tea and stimulant soft drinks which deplete your energy reserves.

Heal well

Do not underestimate the effects of minor illness on energy burn. Fever uses energy and suppresses your appetite to encourage rest. Fighting this natural mechanism depletes your energy stores and increases the time it takes to heal.

Adapt with age

At different times of our lives we have different energy needs. As we grow older our energy burn decreases and daily calorie needs reduce. Understanding our varying energy requirements helps to maintain good health at any age.

Digest food

Ten per cent of our daily energy is used for digesting, absorbing and metabolizing food. Allow yourself some quiet time after eating for digestion, and avoid high protein meals when you need to keep alert.

Gauge your needs

Do not underestimate your energy needs if your day consists of sustained, physical effort. Standing for a long period can use up as much energy as a short burst of extreme physical activity – energy burn depends on time as well as exertion.

Nature's best

To build a durable house, you need good foundations. To build a strong and healthy body, you need good food. As everything we eat is either a plant or comes from an animal that eats plants, it follows that the foundation of good food is healthy plants. And every gardener knows that healthy plants grow in healthy soil. So, if we really care about our food and health, our first concern should be for the health of the land.

The problem is that most people simply regard food as something bought in the grocery store or supermarket. Although we may feel uncomfortable about antibiotic, hormone and pesticide residues, diseased cattle, food irradiation, genetically modified crops and the hundred-and-one other "food safety scares" that seem to be part of modern living, our relationship with the farmer and the land is now so distant that we often feel powerless to create change. But once we remember that food production and supply systems depend on consumer demand, it becomes clear that we *can* make a difference by choosing carefully which produce we buy.

Organic fruit and vegetables, which have been grown using traditional, pesticide-free methods with natural fertilizers, contain more nutrients and also often taste better than mass-market produce. So every time we eat organic, locally or regionally grown, fresh, seasonal, minimally processed and minimally packaged energy foods, we put back one more brick in the pyramid of health. Next time you shop at the supermarket, bear in mind that by "going organic" you are setting in motion a knock-on effect that will produce healthier soil, healthier plants, healthier animals and, ultimately, healthier people.

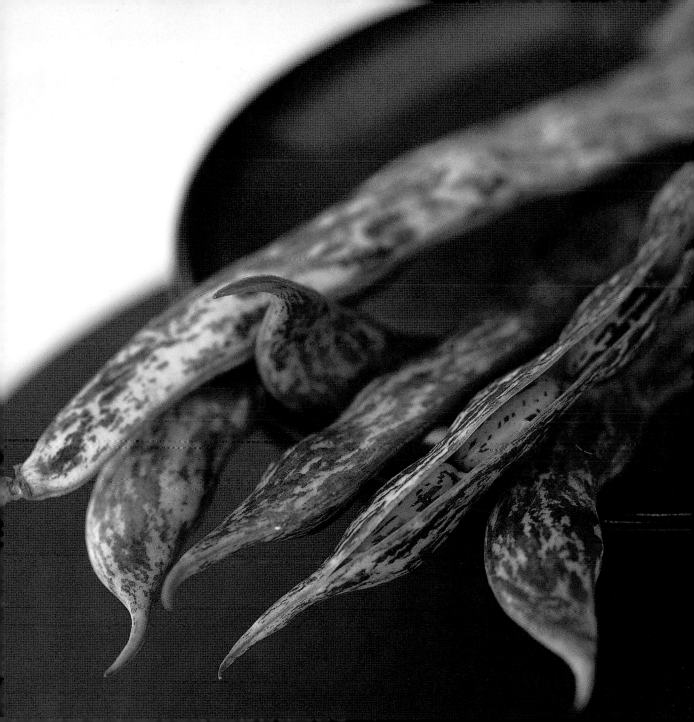

The inner sea

the essence of life

Water. It surrounds and protects us before we are born, our bodies are three-quarters made from it and our digestion and metabolism depend on it. Without it there would be no life on our planet.

In the migration from the sea to dry land, living organisms solved the physiological challenge posed by their new environment by incorporating the ocean within their tissues. Salt water became the internal medium in which materials could be transported around the body. It provided structure and solidity to cells, lubrication to moving parts, protection to delicate organs, and a way of maintaining a constant internal environment in the face of an ever-changing external world.

As evolutionary inheritors of this inner sea, we too depend on water for life and wellbeing. Our brains are 70 per cent water, our blood 60 per cent, and even our bones are 30 per cent. An "average" 155-lb man is made up of about 94 pints of water – 63 pints inside his cells, 25 pints filling the spaces between his tissues and 6 pints in his blood plasma.

Saliva, tears, sweat, bile, gastric juices, pancreatic fluid, cerebrospinal fluid, seminal fluid, amniotic fluid and urine all contain a high proportion of water, and the evaporation of water from the skin in the form of sweat helps to keep us cool in hot weather. The water balance in our body is closely involved in our temperature control system. In cold weather, our sweat reflex shuts down, allowing the heat from our circulation to maintain a constant internal body temperature. As the poet and philosopher J. W. von Goethe wrote: "All is born of water, and upheld by water too."

Energy juices revitalize and replenish the inner sea by ensuring that the body has access not only to the water but also to the essential nutrients it needs in a form that is easy to absorb and, just as importantly, to enjoy. Juices also encourage the elimination of metabolic wastes from our bodies. Making juices a regular part of our diet is a major step toward long-term health and vitality.

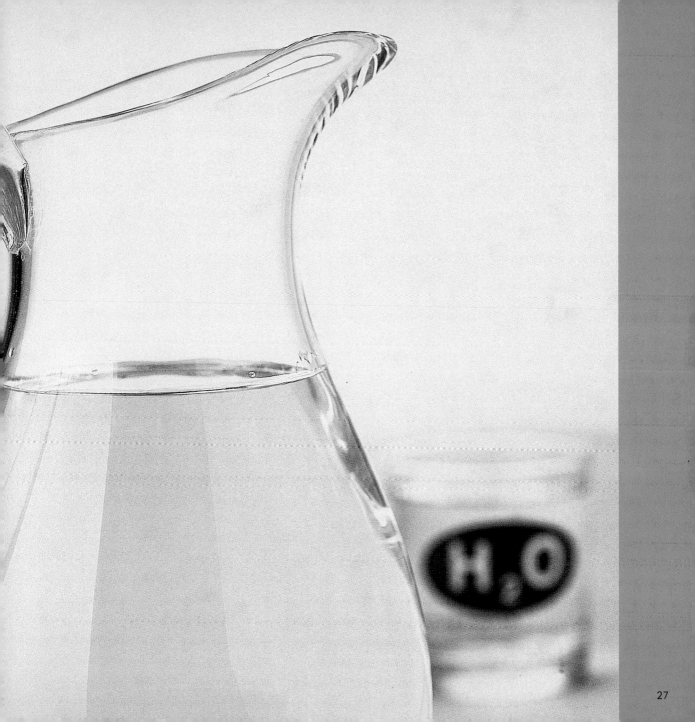

Pure and simple

What, when and how much do we need to drink for perfect health? Some natural medicine practitioners suggest that a proper diet does away with the need to drink extra fluids, while others prescribe strict restrictions on the amount we can drink. But the wisdom of most ancient healing traditions, backed up by the evidence of modern science, is that we should drink little and often throughout the day. This way, we enhance the performance of our mind and body, and avoid the build-up of toxic metabolites in our tissues.

When we are very busy, we often neglect the quiet voice of thirst. As a result, we drink too little and drinking becomes a passive activity rather than a positive contribution to health. We may abandon water and natural juices in favor of "convenient" soft drinks, containing refined sugar or caffeine. Symptoms of dehydration – a dry mouth, tiredness, irritability, concentration loss, infrequent urination, dark urine, and constipation – are accepted as a part of life.

We are constantly losing water from our bodies by evaporation when we sweat, and from our breath when we exhale. Water is also excreted in our urine and feces. If this water is not replaced, the volume of circulating plasma (which carries oxygen and nutrients to our tissues) decreases, waste in our blood becomes more concentrated, and physical and mental abilities deteriorate.

So what does this mean in practice? First, remember that drinking is healthy. Plants and animals all need water. Second, drink about 3 pints of pure water a day, including a small glass of water first thing in the morning and last thing at night to help keep your system running smoothly. (Drink a little water with your meals if you like, but avoid "washing down" food.) Third, exchange black tea and coffee and manufactured soft drinks for herb teas, tisanes and fresh fruit and vegetable juices, which will nourish and detoxify your body and so give you extra energy. And remember to taste what you drink – savor the flavors before you swallow.

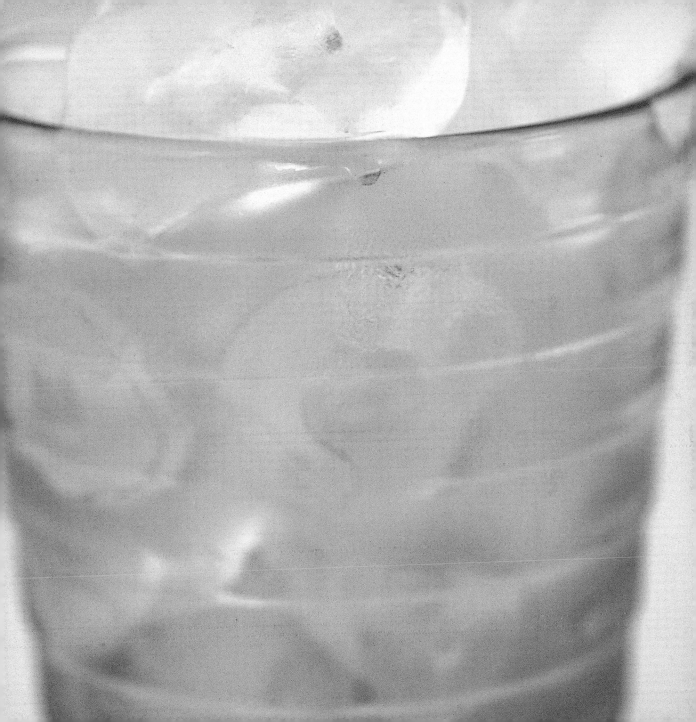

Natural cure

juices for self-healing

In 1958, in his seminal book *A Cancer Therapy*, Dr Max Gerson wrote: "It [is becoming] more and more important that organically grown fruit and vegetables will be, and must be, used for the protection against degenerative disease and the prevention of cancer." But it is only now that we are beginning to understand the mechanisms by which plants promote our health and wellbeing.

International research has shown conclusively that increasing our consumption of fresh fruit and vegetables has a massive impact on our capacity to resist disease. From the prevention of cancer, heart disease and diabetes to protecting us from diverticulitis, hypertension, hemorrhoids and gallstones, a diet rich in plant food is an inexpensive, practical way to avoid illness and increase vitality. This is because fresh fruits and vegetables contain phytochemicals – naturally occurring substances produced by plants to protect themselves from disease and insect damage – which have powerful, beneficial effects on human health (see p.33).

Energy juices, such as those in this book, offer the maximum opportunity to benefit from phytochemicals with minimum time and effort. As the juices are mostly based on raw ingredients, they also provide a concentrated source of the vitamins, minerals and trace elements that we need for peak performance. By using organic ingredients we avoid chemical pollution and ensure maximum nourishment as we drink.

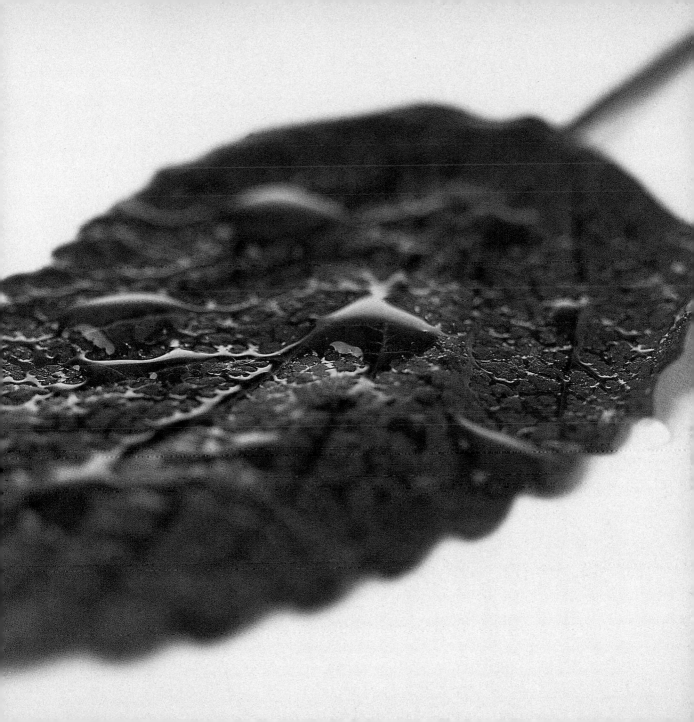

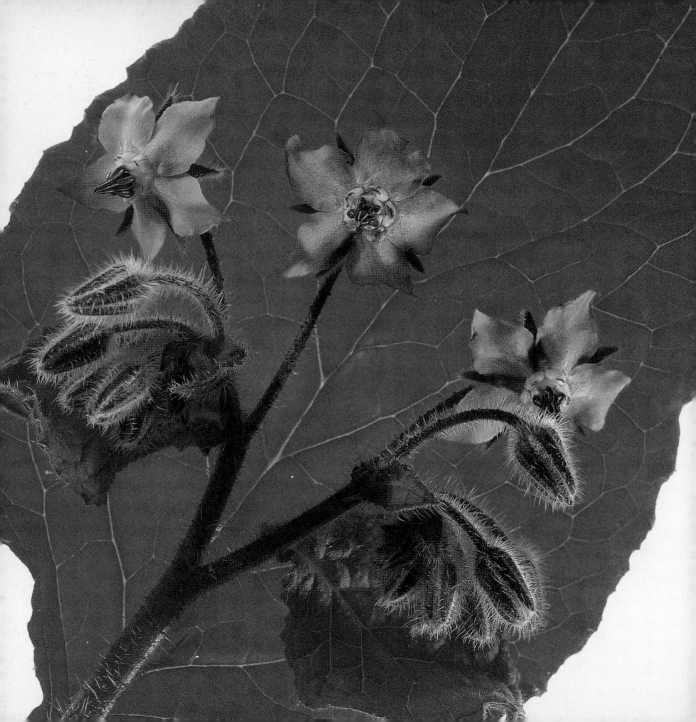

Phytochemicals
nature's health protectors

allium compounds stimulate antioxidants; destroy bacteria.

anthrocyanins are dark-colored, antioxidant chemicals in red grapes, blueberries and cranberries. May reduce the "stickiness" of blood platelets and help prevent blood clots.

carotenoids help prevent the formation of cancer cells and may be important in determining our lifespan. They are found in yellow and orange fruits and vegetables.

coumarins stop the formation of tumors.

dithiolthyones help to maintain the health of cell membranes and the structure of chromosomes.

flavonoids are antioxidant chemicals which inhibit cancer-cell growth and may help prevent hypertension.

glucosinolates and indoles support the detoxifying action of the liver.

isoflavones help control cell growth rates.

limonene is a detoxifying chemical found in citrus fruits.

phenols inhibit the production of carcinogens.

protease inhibitors help to stop the spread of tumor cells into surrounding tissues.

saponins may help control blood cholesterol and reduce the growth rate of some tumor cells. They are found in soy products and anti-inflammatory herbs, such as chickweed.

sterols improve the health of cell membranes and may protect against colonic cancer.

thiocyanates protect DNA and block carcinogen activity.

Natural healers
the health-enhancing properties of six juice giants

beet Often called the "vitality plant", beet is rich in folate, iron and magnesium. Used to relieve all chronic illnesses, particularly those of the blood and immune system, it may also help the body to fight cancer. (Note: if you consume a lot of beet, your feces and urine may develop a reddish tint. This is harmless and will disappear if you reduce your intake of the food.)

carrot Extremely rich in carotenes (and a good source of fiber and chromium), carrots are traditionally used to treat digestive upsets and worms. Beta-carotene may help prevent cancer of the lungs, cervix and gastro-intestinal tract. Carrot is also thought to boost immunity, making it useful in treating chronic viral infections such as herpes simplex.

cranberry Long used to relieve urinary-tract infections, cranberry juice contains a phytochemical that prevents harmful bacteria from sticking to the bladder wall. In addition, it has powerful antioxidant effects which may improve cardiovascular health and help to prevent cancer.

red grape As well as containing anthrocyanins, which may decrease the stickiness of blood platelets and reduce the likelihood of blood clots, red grape juice also contains a compound called reservatol, which lowers blood cholesterol and may inhibit the formation of cancer cells.

orange and grapefruit The high vitamin C content of these fruits helps to maintain healthy blood cells and may increase resistance to viral infections. Vitamin C may also help to lower blood cholesterol and protect against breast cancer. (Note: the vitamin C in fresh-pressed citrus juice deteriorates rapidly – only press as much as you are going to drink straightaway.)

Clear as crystal

energy juices for brain power

Nutrition has important effects on the mind, and changes in neuro-transmitter levels caused by food can have a profound influence on mood and behavior. For example, if we eat plenty of fresh fruit and vegetables, we increase the ratio of carbohydrate to protein in our diet. This in turn increases the availability of tryptophan, the amino acid that our brain uses to make a neuro-transmitter called serotonin. Low levels of serotonin are known to be a cause of depression, so eating more healthily can be a highly effective safeguard against a depressed mood.

Energy juices are particularly useful for keeping the brain active and alert because even though the brain comprises only 2 per cent of our total body weight, it is incredibly active metabolically and uses 20 per cent of the oxygen we breathe to sustain itself. This, plus the fact that it can use only simple glucose as "fuel", means that the brain has a particular need for energy and micronutrients in order to work efficiently. Drinking freshly made organic fruit and vegetable juices is a perfect way to ensure that we get top-quality nutrition where it is needed most – fast!

Energy juices also help to guard against the decrease in mental clarity and efficiency that minor nutritional deficiencies may cause. For example, a low intake of vitamin B_1 may result in poor sleep, restlessness, fatigue and changes in mood. A lack of vitamin B_6 is linked with anxiety, depression and premenstrual tension. Low levels of folate and vitamin C may cause a lowering of mood and other psychological disturbances.

A change in body potassium levels (caused by excessive intakes of tea, coffee and alcohol) leads to apathy and lethargy; and deficiencies in zinc and magnesium can lead to irritability, mood swings, poor appetite, anxiety, insomnia and fatigue. Low iron intake causes tiredness and weakness and interferes with our ability to take in new information. Insufficient chromium increases the likelihood of fatigue, anxiety and depression related to low blood-sugar levels.

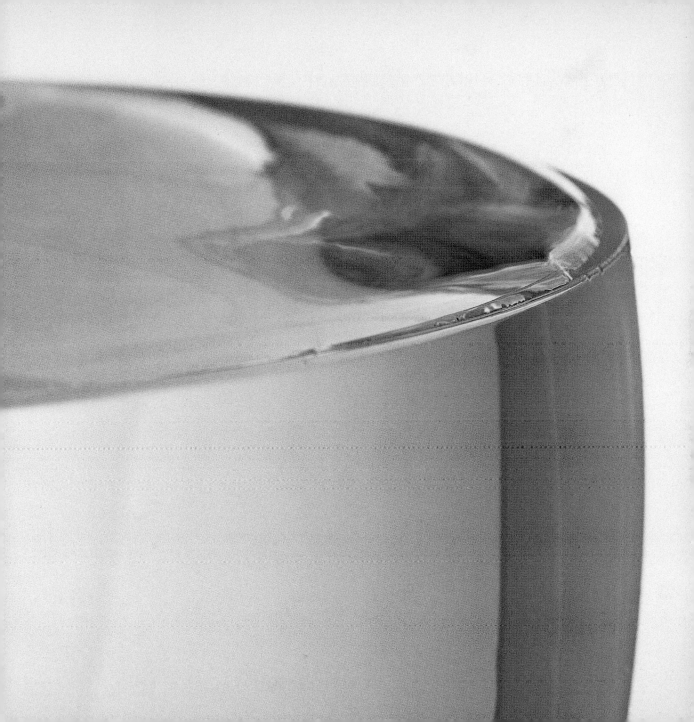

24-hour detox

cleanse the body, clear the mind

Detoxing will make you feel lighter in yourself, and help to reduce your susceptibility to stress and illness. But the most immediate and striking improvement you will notice after detoxifying is that you will have much more energy. Other benefits include shinier hair, clearer skin, better sleep, improved digestion, sweeter breath, a more sensitive sense of smell, a clearer brain and a calmer state of mind.

Detoxification involves using all available resources for body healing and regeneration. Every now and then, use the following, simple, 24-hour plan to give your digestive system a rest and to help your body to rid itself of accumulated toxins. Choose a day when you can be sure of peace and quiet, and have a comfortable, warm environment in which you can sleep as much as you wish.

The day before starting your detox, cut out all stimulants (tea, coffee, chocolate, tobacco, alcohol and so on); sugar (candy, cakes, sodas); meat and dairy products; and processed foods.

On the day, follow the menu plan as shown opposite. Take as much rest as you can, keep warm and drink pure water, little and often. Spend some time outside in the fresh air, but keep any activities gentle.

After your 24-hour detox, stay off stimulants and do not eat processed foods for a week. Take stock of your diet and listen to your body – it knows instinctively which foods are good for you and which are not.

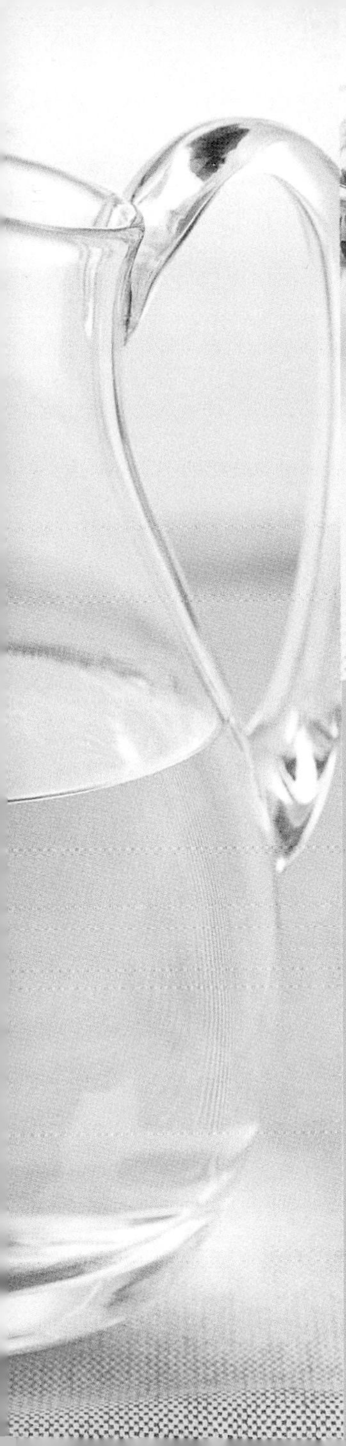

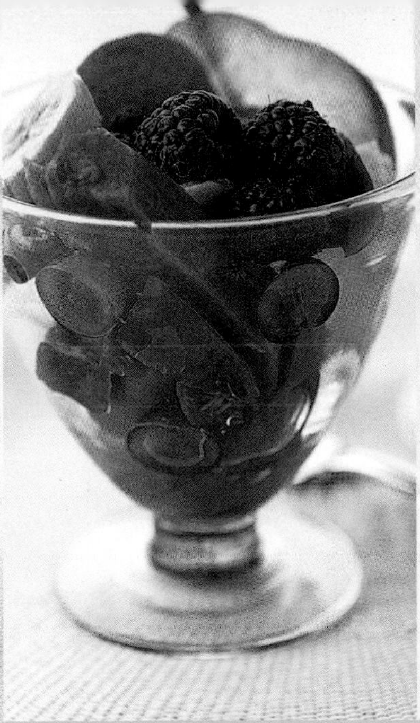

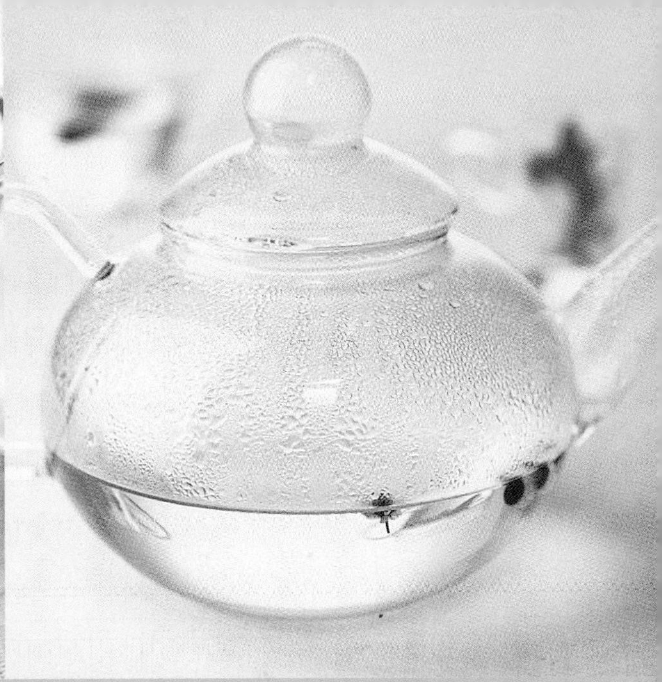

Detox menu plan

Breakfast
Fresh fruit salad (see p.75)

Mid-morning
1 cup nettle tea

Lunch
$1/4$ melon, followed by fruit
salad comprising:
1 thick slice pineapple, chunked
1 sliced banana
1 apple, cored and chopped
1 pear, cored and chopped
6 grapes, halved and pipped
5 tablespoons unsweetened fruit juice

Mid-afternoon
1 cup thyme tea (see p.130)

Dinner
$1/2$ papaya
1 mango

After dinner
1 cup camomile tea

Note: We do not recommend that you do
the 24-hour detox during menstruation, nor
if you are pregnant or breast feeding. If you
are taking medication, check with your
doctor before following the plan.

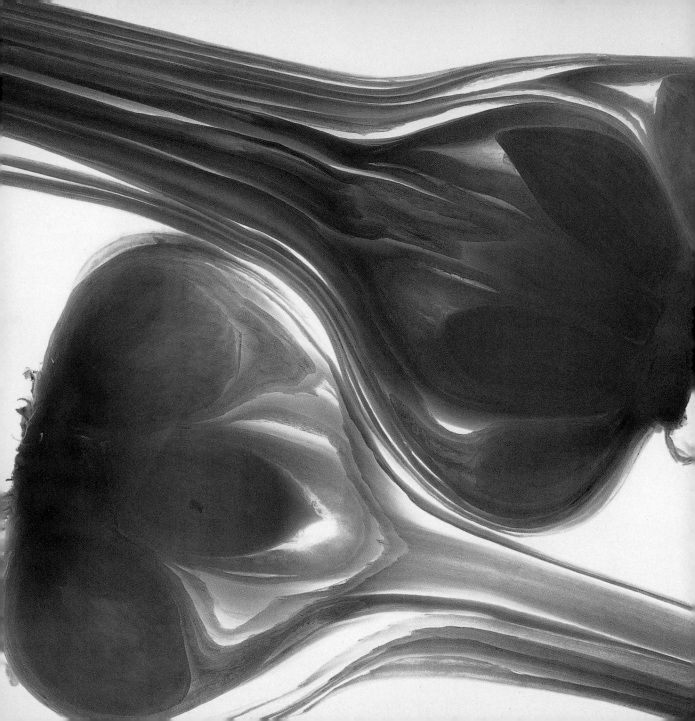

chapter two

Foods for life

Energy foods are the foundations of health and vitality. They fall into natural groups which supply the different nutrients we need to provide an energy-rich diet.

As the level of energy that we need on a daily basis varies depending on our activity, our age, and the type of metabolism we have, it makes sense to base our diet on those foods which optimize our energy output accordingly – fresh fruit and vegetables, pulses, pasta and wholegrain bread. In the following pages we take a look at the most important food groups and learn how to get the best out of them.

Fruit and vegetables

nature's own convenience foods

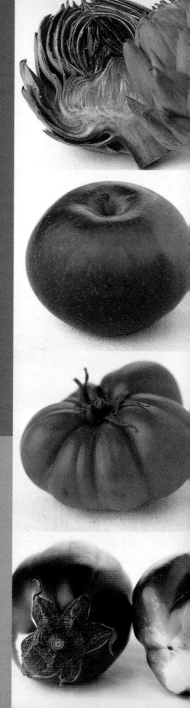

Fruit and vegetables are our link to the vital energies of the sun and the earth. The plants that bear them use sunlight to make the starches which are our primary source of complex carbohydrates, and an important supplier of energy to our bodies. And fresh fruit and vegetables are full of proteins, oils and minerals, which help us to share in the goodness in the soil. When our diet is rich in such foods, we fulfil our nutritional needs without having to take supplements.

Nature's own energy foods, fruit and vegetables are delicious, relatively inexpensive and can be enjoyed raw or cooked at any time, with a minimum of preparation.

Here are some good reasons to include fresh fruit and vegetables in your diet.

✪ Fruit and vegetables are naturally high in fiber and low in cholesterol, as well as being rich in polyunsaturates, and essential amino and fatty acids. They contain no harmful saturated fats or trans-fatty acids.

✪ It is now proven beyond doubt that eating more fruit and vegetables protects our bodies against most cancers.

✪ Eating natural fruit and vegetable fiber reduces the chances of suffering from heart problems and bowel disease.

✪ Fruit and vegetables contain a cocktail of health-enhancing phytochemicals (see p.33), which play a crucial role in our metabolism and boost our immune system.

✪ Eating at least five portions of fruit and vegetables daily can help us to shrug off minor ailments.

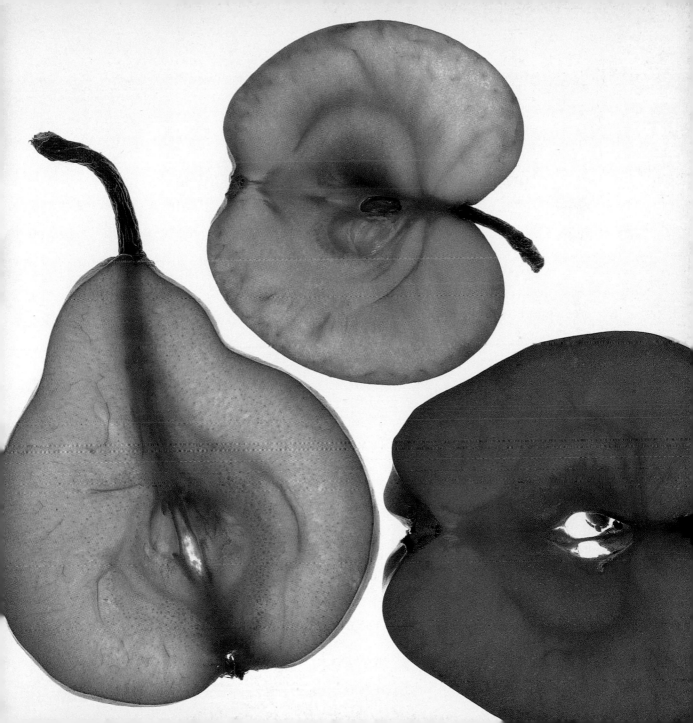

Raw energy
eating it like it is

Human beings are the only creatures who do not eat most of their food fresh and raw. Although cooking reduces the amount of time we spend eating – cooked food requires less chewing – it alters the chemical make-up of food and can destroy essential nutrients. Vitamins A, C and E (important antioxidants), thiamin and folic acid are damaged or destroyed by heat. The structure of amino acids, such as lysine, can also be changed by the cooking process, with the result that they cannot be absorbed by our bodies.

Eating some raw food every day offers many health benefits. It helps us maintain a natural water balance, reduces our salt intake, and ensures that we obtain the maximum benefit from the large variety of cancer-protective phytochemicals contained in fresh fruit and vegetables. Raw food diets can improve our resistance to minor illnesses such as colds and 'flu, and also help us deal more effectively with chronic conditions such as arthritis and diabetes.

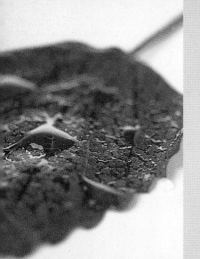

As it is not always practical or convenient to eat raw food, here are some tips to help minimize vitamin and mineral loss when cooking fresh, organic vegetables.

✪ When cleaning vegetables, keep washing to the minimum that is consistent with good hygiene.

✪ Do not pre-soak vegetables, or start cooking them in cold water. Put them straight into boiling water or steam them.

✪ Cook vegetables as lightly as possible – they should be firm and tender, not soggy.

✪ Make sauces and gravies with the vegetable cooking-water so that you can benefit from any vitamins and minerals that they have lost to the water.

✪ Try shallow-frying chopped vegetables in a little oil, then cooking them in a covered pan with a little water – a great way to preserve both flavor and nutrients.

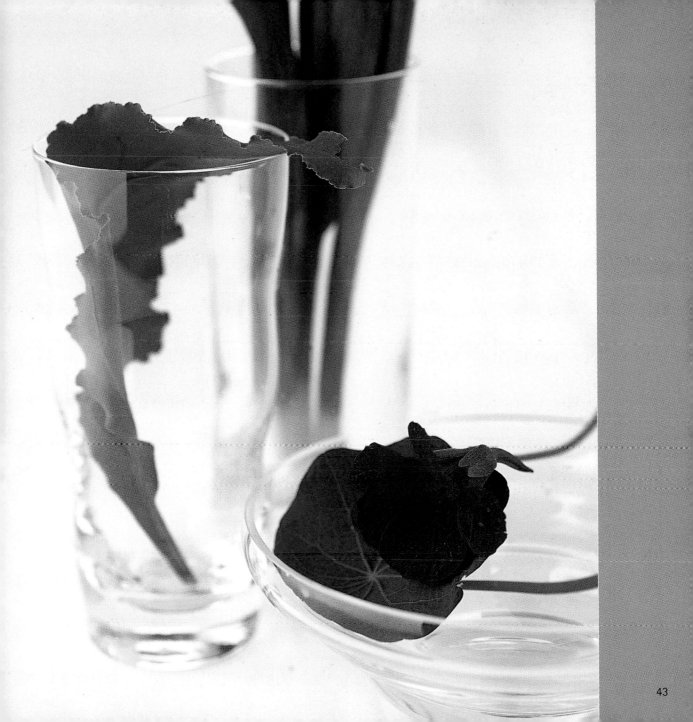

Cereal grains

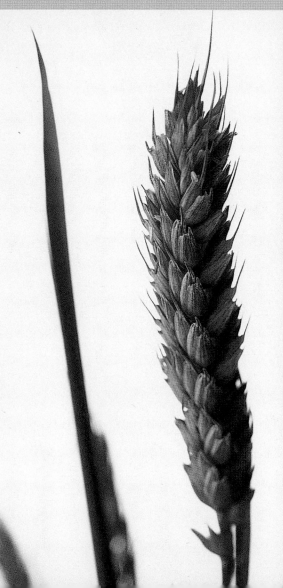

The main source of energy and protein for people in the world today is cereal grains. Here is a guide to the most important varieties.

Rice has been a staple food in the East for more than 5,000 years. De-hulled but unpolished, it is a great source of protein, energy, fiber and B-vitamins. "Wild rice" is a native American grain, unrelated to common rice, but also highly nutritious.

Oats are a high-protein cereal, rich in iron and soluble fiber. By lowering the body's blood cholesterol levels they reduce the risk of coronary heart disease. Naturopaths value oats' ability to ease stress and soothe tired nerves. Uniquely, they lose little of their nutritional value when commercially processed into flakes or oatmeal.

Maize (also known as corn) originated in the Americas and was brought to Europe by the explorer Christopher Columbus (1451–1506). It has a particular claim to be called an "energy food" as it yields a large energy-rich crop in a small area of land. Dishes combining maize, beans and green vegetables are especially nutritious.

Buckwheat was first grown in China but is now popular in central and Eastern Europe. Its traditional reputation for being "warming and drying" makes it a good source

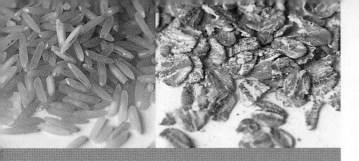

of energy in winter. Kasha, made from buckwheat groats roasted briefly in a dry pan then cooked in vegetable stock with a bayleaf until soft, makes a nourishing and tasty alternative to rice.

Quinoa and amaranth are ancient Andean plants that thrive in mountain climates. Among the most nutritious of all grains and rich in protein and minerals, they can be used to add variety to savory casseroles, breakfast cereals and cookies.

Millet is a staple food in many parts of Africa, China and India, and the dietary cornerstone of the healthy and long-lived Hunza people of north-west Pakistan. Now neglected in the West, it is a delicious alternative to oats in oatmeal, and is a good source of magnesium and iron.

Rye was the main bread-making ingredient in medieval northern Europe, and enjoys a long-standing "muscle-making" reputation in Scandinavia, Germany and Eastern Europe. Traditional "sour-dough" rye bread can turn a simple sandwich into a nutritious meal, and rye crispbreads are a source of protein as well as energy.

Wheat is the world's most popular grain, accounting for more than 25 per cent of global cereal production. A very versatile foodstuff, it is used to make bread, pasta, couscous and tabouleh.

Peas, beans and lentils

Peas, beans and lentils (also known collectively as pulses or legumes) have a history stretching back at least 7,000 years, and were known to civilizations from ancient Egypt to Mexico. They are packed with top-quality protein, complex carbohydrates, fiber, vitamins and minerals so they are extremely satisfying yet have a negligible fat content. Their ability to lower blood cholesterol helps to prevent heart disease, and the slow way in which they are digested and absorbed makes them an ideal food for diabetics. Peas, beans and lentils are inexpensive, versatile and easy to store.

Here are some ways to make the most of these natural energy boosters.

✪ When buying dried pulses, look for a rich color and regular shape. Choose a reliable organic supplier and avoid old stock.

✪ Pulses should be cooked until they are soft and tender. Add a small potato to the cooking water of dried pulses that require pre-soaking – it makes them easier to digest. Do not add salt until just before serving.

✪ Help your digestive system to adapt to eating pulses. Start off with split peas, dhals and lentils, or try some bottled (pre-cooked) organic, lima beans or garbanzo beans.

✪ Pulses are highly concentrated, high-protein foods best enjoyed in moderation. 1–3 oz dry weight per day is ample.

✪ Soy bean, mung bean and garbanzo bean sprouts are delicious additions to salads, adding vital nutrients as well as flavor.

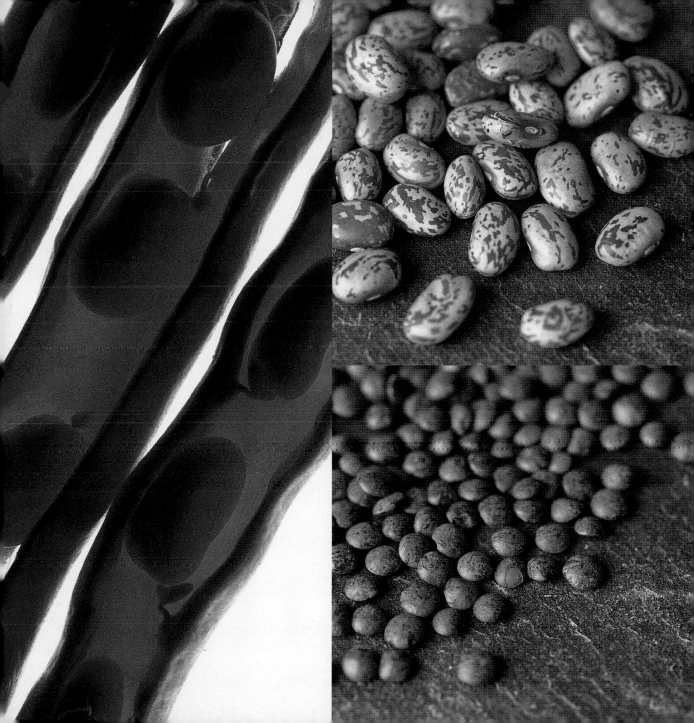

Pasta
ideal fuel for action

The earliest surviving written reference to pasta dates from the 13th-century, but depictions have been found in Etruscan murals dating from as early as c.400BC. Today the peoples of Italy and northern China eat pasta as a staple food, while all over the world it has become a popular meal for anyone wanting a quick-cooking and nutritious source of energy.

Durum wheat – the traditional basis of Italian pasta – is particularly high in the protein gluten, which makes it easy to form into the many shapes beloved of pasta connoisseurs: spaghetti, lasagne, penne, macaroni and fettucine, to name but a few. The density of durum wheat means that it is digested more slowly than other wheat products, releasing a steady flow of energy into the body.

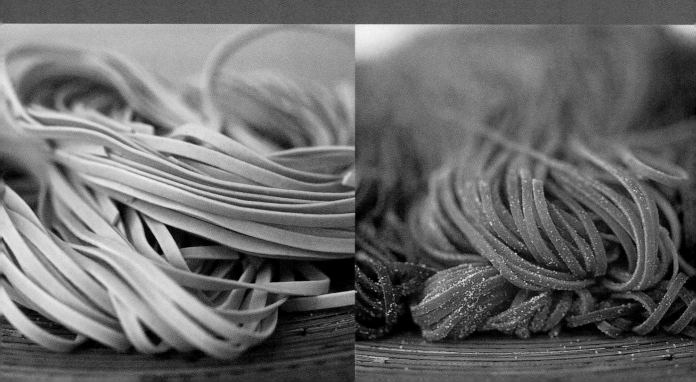

Here are some variations on the pasta theme which you can use to add new flavors and textures to your meals.

✪ Powdered beet, spinach, tomatoes, carrots and herbs can be mixed with durum wheat flour to enhance the visual and nutritional quality of pasta, as well as the taste.

✪ Wholegrain pasta – durum wheat flour mixed with other wheat flours – is richer in vitamins and heavier in texture than other pasta. It has a distinctive, "nutty" flavor which is sometimes considered an acquired taste.

✪ Noodles enriched with amaranth or quinoa (see p.45) are highly nutritious, and lesser-known pastas such as *udon* (Japanese rice and wheat spaghetti) and *soba* (made with buckwheat, wheat and herbs) make an exotic change.

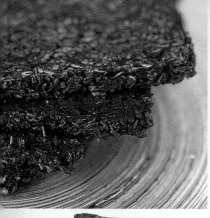
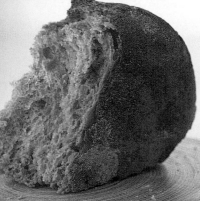
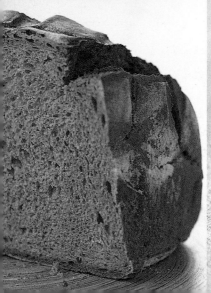
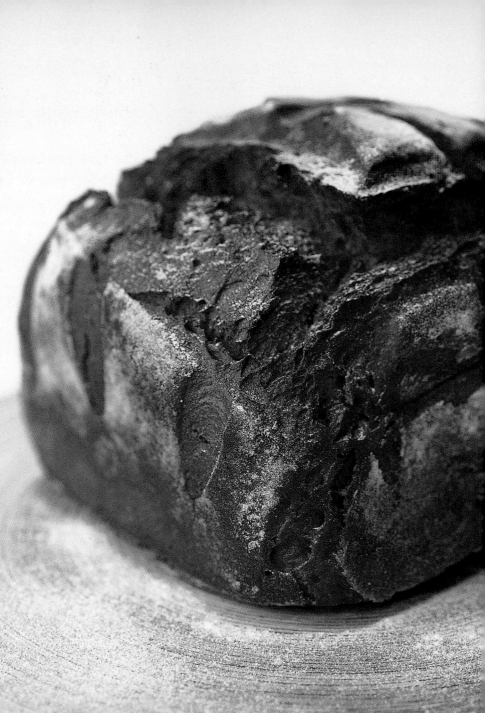

Breads
sustaining the world

A symbol of life and abundance, bread has been at the heart of human nutrition for more than 15,000 years. It is eaten around the world in a multitude of forms ranging from baguettes to bagels, pumpernickel to soda bread, chapatis to tortillas. It is a vital supplier of energy, protein, fiber, B-vitamins, iron, calcium and trace elements. Bread can be made from any cereal, but the flour of wheat is particularly suitable as it contains gluten, a protein that becomes sticky when mixed with water. The gluten traps the gas produced by fermenting yeast inside the batter and makes the bread rise.

To say that home-made, wholegrain bread is healthiest is almost a cliché, but here are some facts that show it is based on truth.

✪ White flours are "enriched" with vitamins and minerals, but enriching does not replace the vitamin B_6, vitamin E, folic acid, pantothenic acid, magnesium and zinc lost during the refining process.

✪ Commercially produced "added bran" flours are less digestible than traditional stoneground and sifted flours in which the non-nutritious, outer covering of the wheat grain, known as the "bee's wing", has been removed.

✪ To cut costs and production times, industrial bread manufacturers use a process involving chemicals and mechanical mixers, instead of traditional kneading and rising.

✪ White loaves typically contain only half the fiber of their wholegrain counterparts.

✪ Bread consumption in industrialized countries has decreased by half in the past hundred years. During the same period, heart disease, cancer, and bowel problems have shown a dramatic increase. Eating wholegrain bread helps safeguard long-term health and adds flavor and substance to any diet.

51

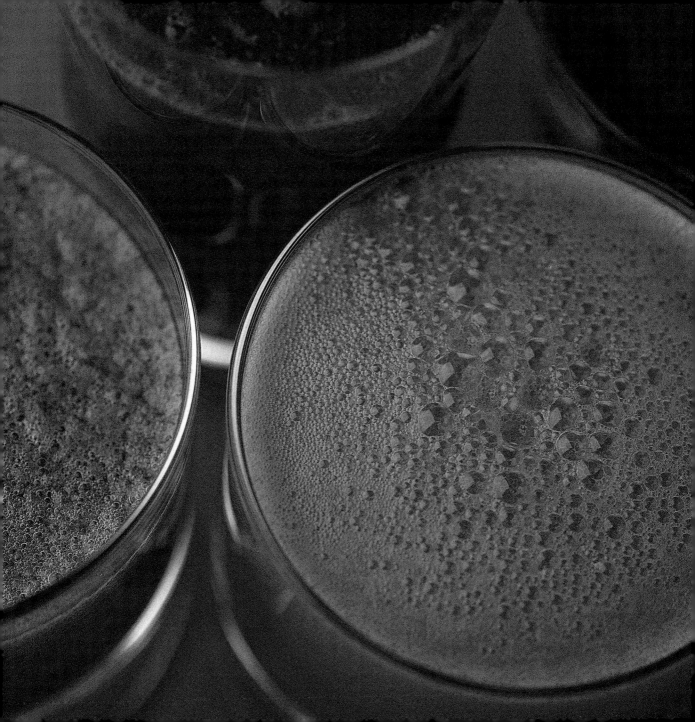

chapter three

Liquid energy

In the midst of a busy life, freshly made organic juices, shakes, teas, tisanes, cocktails and smoothies can provide a sheet anchor for optimum health.

Fruits, vegetables and other natural foods contain many different nutrients, all providing us with particular benefits. Understanding what is in each ingredient of an energy juice helps us to make the best choice, so that each drink we make will give us optimum health and maximum energy. There is a juice to suit any time of day or any mood. The basic methods for each type of energy juice can be expanded on to create countless delicious juice recipes.

Fresh juices

the best in preventative medicine

In chemical terms, a fresh-pressed juice is simply a mixture of water and plant sugars plus small amounts of oils, vitamins, minerals, amino acids and phytochemicals. But these constituents can have a potent effect, helping us to fight disease and counteracting the harmful effects of medicinal drugs, caffeine, tobacco and food additives.

Fruits and vegetables contain different nutrients in varying amounts so, to help you tailor-make your own energy juices, on pages 57 and 59 we have summarized the major benefits of all the important vitamins, minerals and trace elements, together with a selection of the fruits and vegetables that are most abundant in them. But first, here are some tips on choosing and handling energy juice ingredients:

• Try to find a reliable supplier of fresh organic fruits and vegetables – herbicides, pesticides or other agrochemicals, found in conventionally farmed foods, will be concentrated in a juice, greatly diminishing its benefits and they may even be harmful to your health.

• Fresh vegetables should be firm, colorful and "alive". Bananas should be fully ripe; apricots orange-yellow blushed with pink or red; peaches weighty and fragrant; and oranges and grapefruits smooth. Look for grapes with green stems; unshrivelled guavas; firm lychees; kiwis that are slightly but uniformly soft; sweet-smelling melons and pineapples; and yielding, aromatic mangoes. Avoid strawberries with white tips, cherries that are too pale or too soft, and green paw-paws.

• Fruits and vegetables should be properly cleaned before juicing, but avoid soaking them. When removing skins, peel as finely as possible to preserve vital nutrients.

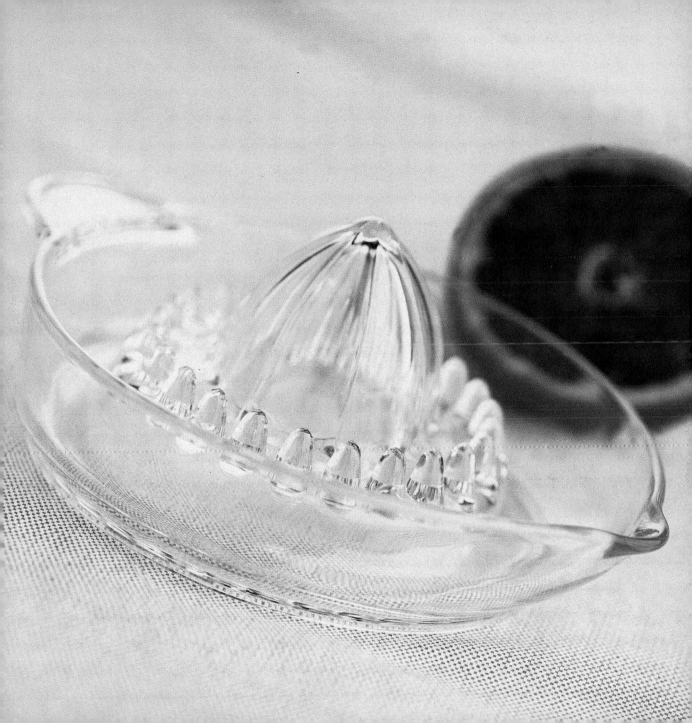

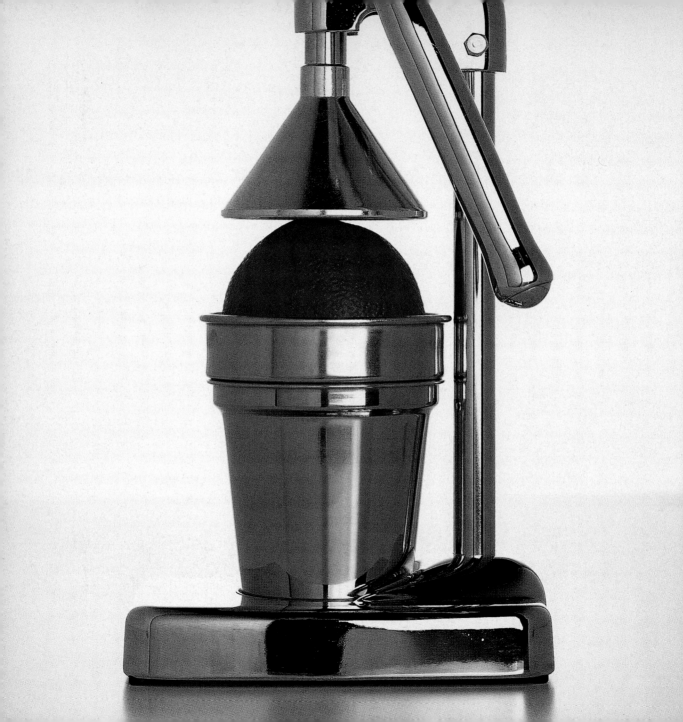

Use this table and the one on p.59 to help you to create your own special juice combinations.

VITAMIN	HEALTH BENEFITS	ENERGY JUICE SOURCES
A	Antioxidant. Keeps skin and vision healthy. Anti-cancer.	Carrots, mangoes, melons, tomatoes.
E	Antioxidant. Good for blood cells, muscles and nervous system. Protects against heart disease and some cancers.	Fresh almond milk, blackberries, filberts.
K	Helps prevent osteoporosis. Ensures normal blood clotting.	Carrots, parsley, strawberries.
C	Antioxidant and anti-allergic. Improves iron absorption and wound healing. Helps immunity and blood-fat levels.	Citrus fruits, guavas, kiwis, mangoes, papayas, peaches, strawberries.
B_1 thiamin	Aids metabolism. Maintains healthy nerves and muscles.	Carrots, oranges.
B_2 riboflavin	Helps energy release from food. Keeps mucous membranes in good condition.	Fresh almond milk, blackcurrants, cherries, cucumbers, grapes.
B_3 niacin	Helps maintain optimum energy levels. Keeps skin and mucous membranes in good condition.	Apples, apricots, bananas, lemons, pears, plums, tomatoes.
B_5 pantothenate	Anti-stress. Helps maintain energy levels. Aids antibody production. Protects against hypertension and allergy.	Honey, tomatoes.
B_6 pyridoxine	Supports nervous system. Aids hemoglobin production. May protect against PMS, asthma, migraine and depression.	Bananas, elderberries, oranges, tomatoes.
Biotin	Maintains condition of skin, hair, sweat glands, nerves and bone marrow. Aids fat metabolism. Encourages appetite.	Fresh almond milk, bananas, redcurrants.
Folate	Aids growth and development of a healthy nervous system.	Apples, beets, carrots, oranges.
B_{12}	Supports growth. Maintains health of the blood, bone marrow and the nervous system.	Fortified soy milk.

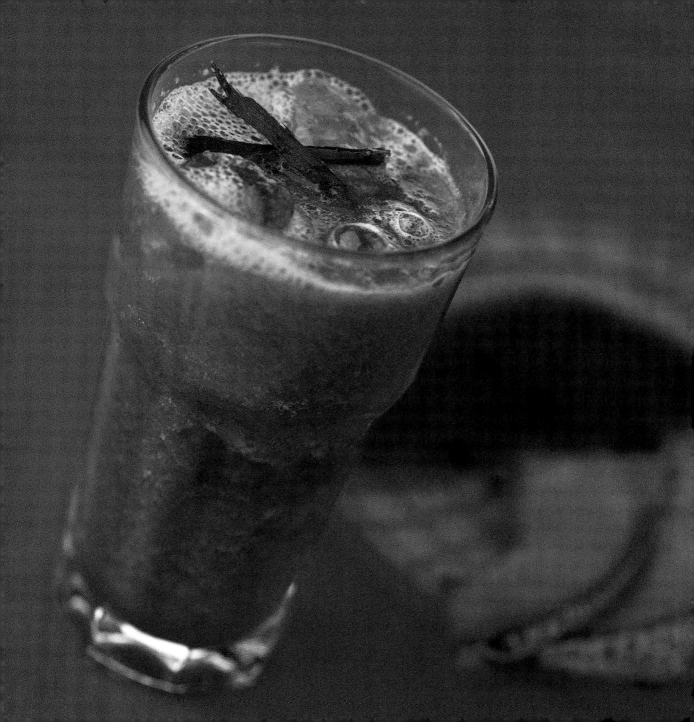

MINERAL	HEALTH BENEFITS	ENERGY JUICE SOURCES
Calcium	Gives structure and strength to bones and teeth. Maintains health of heart, nerve and muscle tissues.	Carrots, lemons, soy milk.
Cobalt	Necessary for the normal action of vitamin B_{12}.	Apricots, cherries.
Copper	Maintains healthy red blood cells and bone and nervous tissue. May help protect against osteoporosis.	Beets, cherries, grapes, honey, melons, oranges, pineapples.
Fluoride	Helps preserve strong bones and teeth.	Apricots, grapes, tomatoes.
Iodine	Supports growth, metabolism and tissue repair.	Garlic, honey, lettuce.
Iron	Enables oxygen transport in the blood and muscles. Maintains energy. Supports nerves. Aids liver function.	Apples, apricots, beets, carrots, honey, pears.
Magnesium	Maintains bones and teeth. Protects against epilepsy, heart disease, hypertension, PMS, osteoporosis, mental illness.	Fresh almond milk, apples, bananas, beets, honey, oranges, soy milk.
Manganese	Helps protein and fat metabolism. Keeps cell membranes healthy. May protect against diabetes, heart disease, epilepsy, cancer and rheumatoid arthritis.	Bananas, blackberries, carrots, celery, dandelion roots, ginger, mulberries, oranges, pears, plums.
Phosphorus	A building block for proteins, carbohydrates and fats. Supports the immune system and helps maintain energy.	Carrots, parsley, prunes, raspberries, soy milk.
Potassium	Keeps heart, muscles and nerves healthy. Boosts energy and strength.	Bananas, honey, soy milk.
Selenium	Antioxidant. Enables red blood cells to function properly.	Celery.
Zinc	Aids wound healing. Maintains skin health. Protects against prostate disorders and mental disturbances. Helps regulate blood fat levels.	Beets, carrots, lettuce, oranges, peaches, tomatoes.

Teas and tisanes

Nourishing, nutrient-packed teas and tisanes made from the leaves, stems, flowers, fruits and seeds of medicinal plants have been used since the beginning of recorded history to improve health and ward off illness. Certain plants, such as mint, are caffeine-free stimulants. Others, such as camomile, aid digestion and help us to relax. Some, such as thyme, boost our natural immunity to infection and disease. All of these plants are gifts from nature – gentle, unadulterated, low-cost natural healers. Most of the plants used in traditional tisanes tend to be hardy and undemanding, and a small back garden or just a sunny windowsill are all you need to grow the ingredients for your favorite plant and herb tea mixtures (see p.130).

Make your teas in a teapot or in a cup with a lid, which will help to preserve the plant's nutritional and medicinal qualities. Use 1 cup of boiling water for each teaspoon of herb. Leave the tea to infuse for about 5 minutes. Here are 5 herbs to try.

✪ **Lemon balm** smells of honey and lemons. It heals, soothes and calms.

✪ Soothing, warming **camomile** is a good aid for the digestive system. It makes an excellent night cap, and is mild enough for children to enjoy.

✪ **Rosemary** stimulates the circulation, and helps to keep the mind clear and alert.

✪ **Sage** can relieve sore throats and reduce sweat, and helps to balance our hormones.

✪ **Yarrow** can ease the symptoms of colds and 'flu, and aids digestion and circulation.

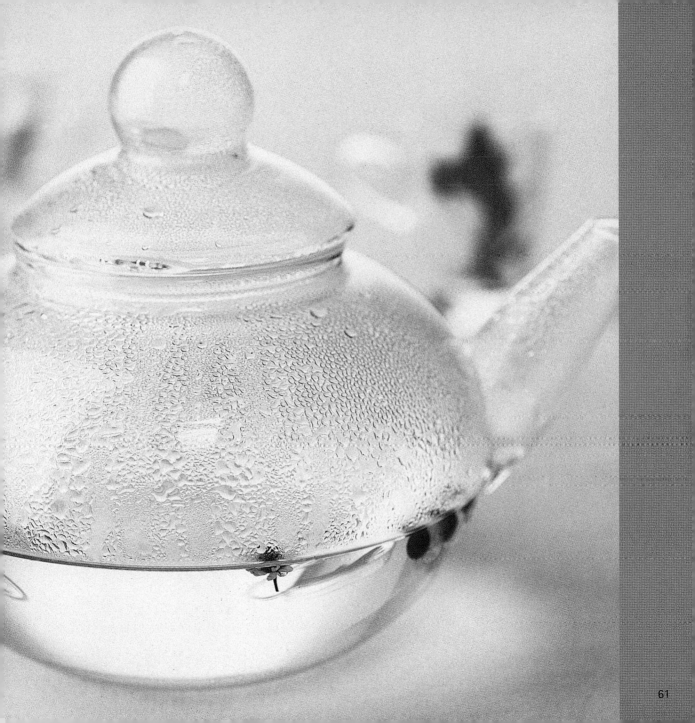

Smoothies and shakes

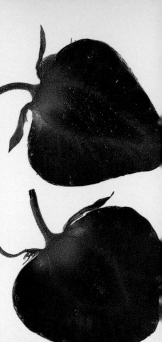

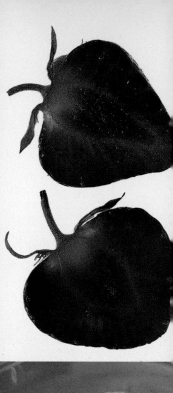

a treat in a glass

Thick, cool, creamy and satisfying, pure fruit smoothies and dairy-free shakes make perfect energy boosters at any time of day, and can even be used as quick and easy substitutes for meals if time is short. They are low in fat and high in essential nutrients.

A smoothie is a mixture of fruits blended with apple, orange or pear juice into a rich, velvety, colorful drink. A shake is a combination of one or two fruits, blended with fresh almond milk or plain organic soy yogurt, and sweetened with a little maple syrup or honey to taste.

Use your favorite fruits, such as organic bananas, raspberries, mangoes or peaches, in any combination you like to make a limitless variety of health-enhancing and delicious drinks.

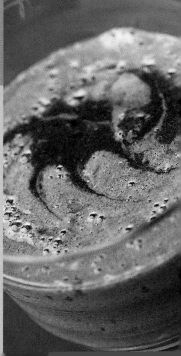

Here are the essentials of what you need to know to make shakes and smoothies:

✪ **Almond milk** Blanch half a cup of shelled almonds in boiling water for 2 minutes. Peel off the brown skins and dry. Grind to a fine powder. Add this to 1 cup water and blend for 2 minutes. Use maple syrup to sweeten. Strain slowly through a fine mesh. In an airtight container, the milk will keep for up to 3 days in the fridge.

✪ **Smoothies** Wash and peel a cupful of your chosen fresh fruit. Add this to 1 cup apple, pear or orange juice. Blend for 30 seconds. Sweeten with maple syrup or honey if necessary. For an ice-cold smoothie, blend a frozen peeled banana with the other fruit.

✪ **Shakes** Blend 1 or 2 chosen fruits (peeled and washed as necessary) and add them to 1 cup fresh almond milk or organic soy yogurt. Add a tablespoon of maple syrup if you like.

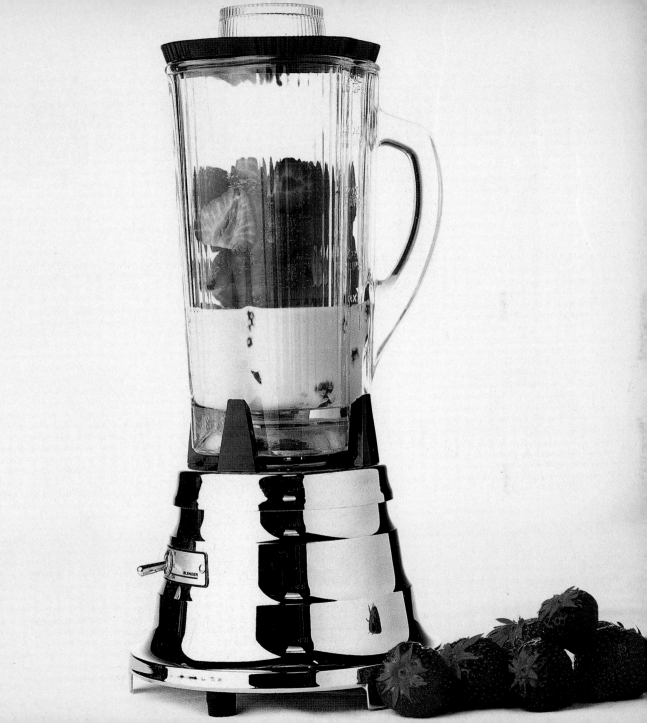

Cocktails

Any combination of brightly colored fluids can be termed a cocktail, so-called because of the drink's resemblance to the multi-colored tail feathers of a farmyard cockerel. We may think of a cocktail as an exotic drink served in bars, at parties or on vacation, but its main purpose is as an apéritif – to stimulate the appetite before a delicious meal. This role is fulfilled perfectly by the clean, light flavors of blended fresh fruit and vegetable juices. What is more, by drinking energy juice cocktails you are at no risk of the negative, long-term health effects of most alcoholic cocktails.

The choice of ingredients for cocktails is limited only by our imagination. There are thousands of exotically named cocktails, alcoholic and non-alcoholic, recorded in books, magazines and the secret notebooks of expert bartenders. Use these drinks as inspiration and experiment with different fruit and vegetable combinations until you find your perfect cocktail.

A colorful, refreshing, non-alcoholic and, above all, healthy fruit-juice cocktail is perhaps a perfect way to end a busy working day and mark the beginning of a relaxed and convivial evening.

Here are some tips to help make energy juice cocktails a treat for the eye and the palate:

✪ Cocktails should be "dry"; in other words, not too sweet. Try different combinations of grapefruit, orange, pineapple, kiwi or mandarin juice sharpened with some freshly squeezed, ripe lemon or lime juice.

✪ For a savory cocktail, try juicing 2 tomatoes, half a peeled cucumber and a stalk of celery and add some lemon juice, gomasio and fresh ground black pepper to taste. For a spicier mix, add a little fresh grated ginger or a sprinkle of cayenne.

✪ Cocktails are best served cold – shake the juice ingredients together with some ice cubes in a cocktail shaker and serve immediately. For added interest, why not make ice cubes with fresh mint or lemon balm leaves "suspended" inside them – just add a leaf to each cube in the ice tray before freezing.

✪ Make your cocktails beautiful to look at. Serve them in elegant or unusual glassware and decorate with fresh fruit slices. You could garnish your drinks with fresh spearmint, lemon balm or cilantro leaves, or a sprinkling of cinnamon or nutmeg.

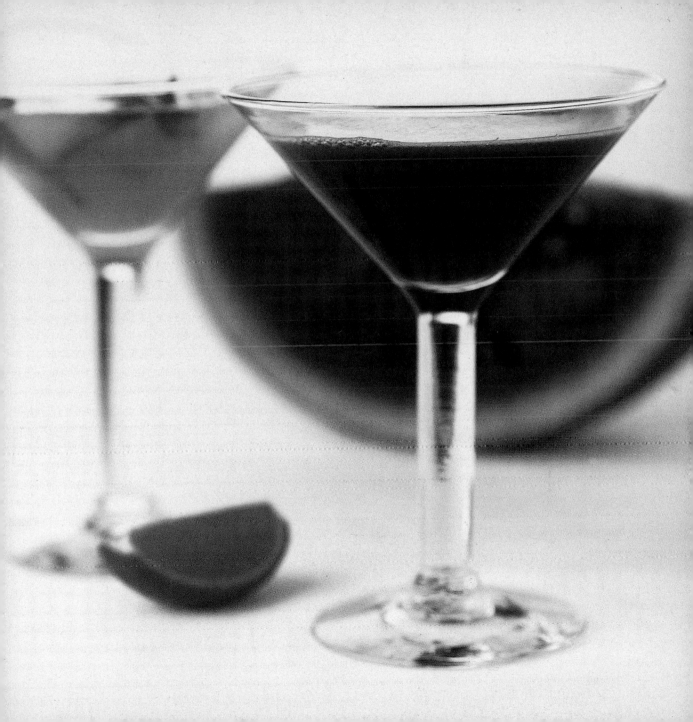

Cordials

distilling the summer

A cordial is a sweet, concentrated juice made from fruits and/or herbs that is diluted with water before drinking. Cordials were invented by monks as a way to preserve medicinal herbs – and to make herbal remedies more palatable to their patients! In his 17th-century medical treatise, the physician and herbalist Nicholas Culpepper said of cordial that it will "... remove all weariness, heat, and tension, of the parts; therefore it is of great service in the depressed state of fevers, fatigue from excesses, and lowness of spirits".

Many liqueurs are derived from early medicinal cordials. Vermouth, for example, is named after the digestive herb wormwood and was originally drunk to aid digestion and stimulate the circulation.

Inexpensive and easy to make, home-prepared cordials preserve the goodness of summer fruits for us to enjoy long into winter.

This basic cordial recipe can be adapted to make many different-flavored cordials, such as blackcurrant, elderberry or redcurrant.

✪ Take 2 lb ripe berries, 2 cups spring water, 2 tablespoons lemon juice, 1 teaspoon citric acid and 1⅓ cups unrefined organic cane sugar.

✪ Rinse the fruit, then place in a pan with the water, lemon juice and citric acid. Cover and heat gently until the berries burst.

✪ Strain the mixture though a cheesecloth, add the sugar and bring the liquid back to a boil. Simmer for 5 minutes.

✪ Skim off any froth, then pour the cordial into sterilized, warm glass bottles (for advice on cleaning glass bottles, refer to books on preserve making, or consult your pharmacist or a supplier of wine-making equipment). Seal and store in a cool, dark place.

✪ Drink diluted with pure water to taste.

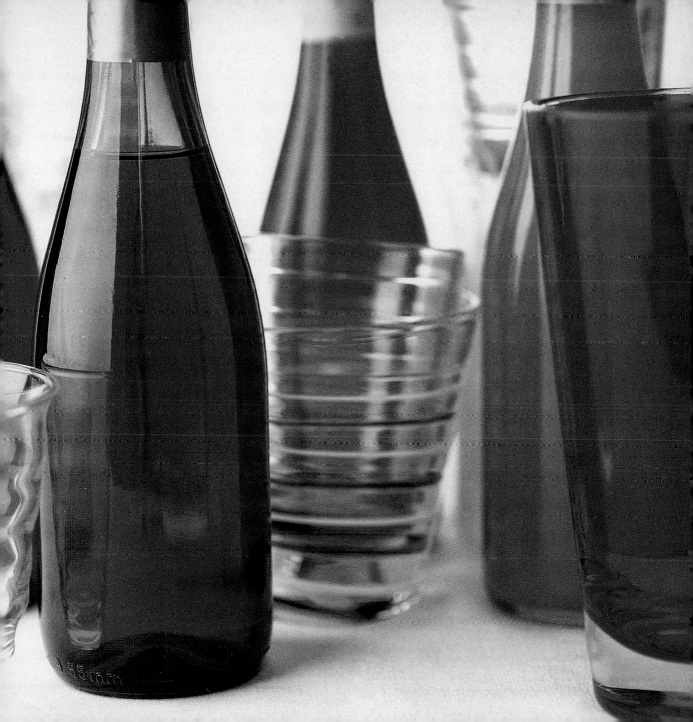

Root drinks

The ubiquitous use of coffee as a pick-me-up and after-meal beverage is regarded by many health experts as a symptom of a stressed-out society, dependent on epinephrine and stimulants and suffering increasingly from burn-out and fatigue. Caffeine-containing drinks give us a quick burst of energy at the expense of our long-term stamina and overall vitality, and may provoke migraine headaches, as well as increasing anxiety and exaggerating the effects of stomach ulcers, hiatus hernia and arthritis.

Root drinks such as dandelion coffee (see p.124) or roasted Belgian endive root (see below) make excellent replacements for traditional coffee. They improve the digestion, support the liver and help detoxify the body. In addition, root drinks have none of the negative effects of caffeine. Dandelion also acts as a general tonic and gentle laxative.

Belgian endive root (*Cichorium intybus*, also known as succory) was used by the Ancient Greeks and Romans to make digestive beverages, and is still a popular substitute for (and addition to) coffee in many parts of Europe. Belgian endive has a distinctive bitter taste, but you can sweeten the coffee with a little honey if you like.

✪ You can buy ready-made roast Belgian endive drinks and blends in good health stores but it is far more fun to grow your own Belgian endive and transform it into a delicious drink. The best varieties are Magdeburg, Brunswick or Witloof.

✪ Belgian endive makes a beautiful addition to any garden, attracting bees and butterflies in the summer. It has bright blue flowers (folk tales hold that they are the tears of a girl weeping for her lover lost at sea). The flowers open and close with such regularity that they can be used as a "floral clock". You can also use Belgian endive as a compass – wherever it grows, the leaves always point north!

✪ To make Belgian endive coffee, lift the roots from established plants in the late fall. Remove any side shoots and top and tail so that each root is approximately 8 in long.

✪ Wash the roots thoroughly and slice thinly. Place in a warm oven, 210–300°F until completely dry.

✪ Dry-fry the dried roots in a heavyweight skillet until they are dark brown in color – this takes about 10 minutes. Allow the roots to cool, then grind them to a fine powder using an electric coffee grinder. Use in the same way as ground coffee.

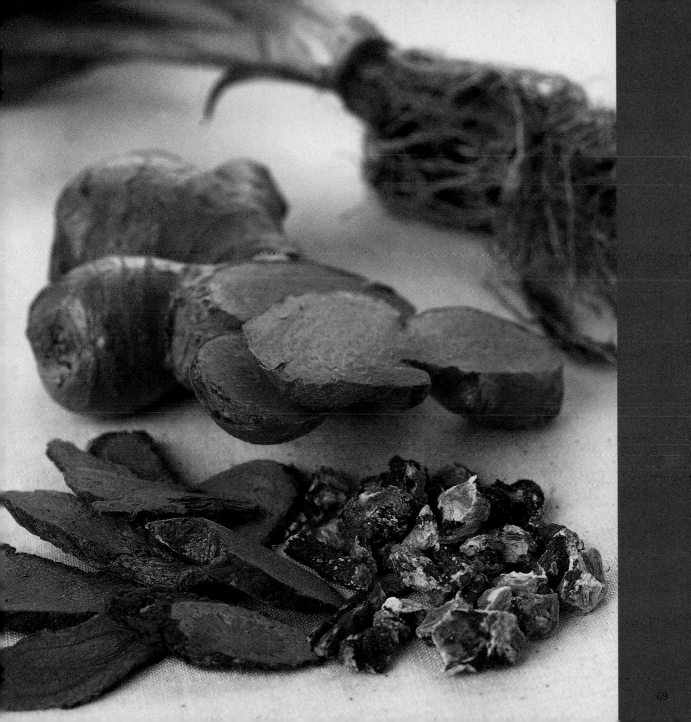

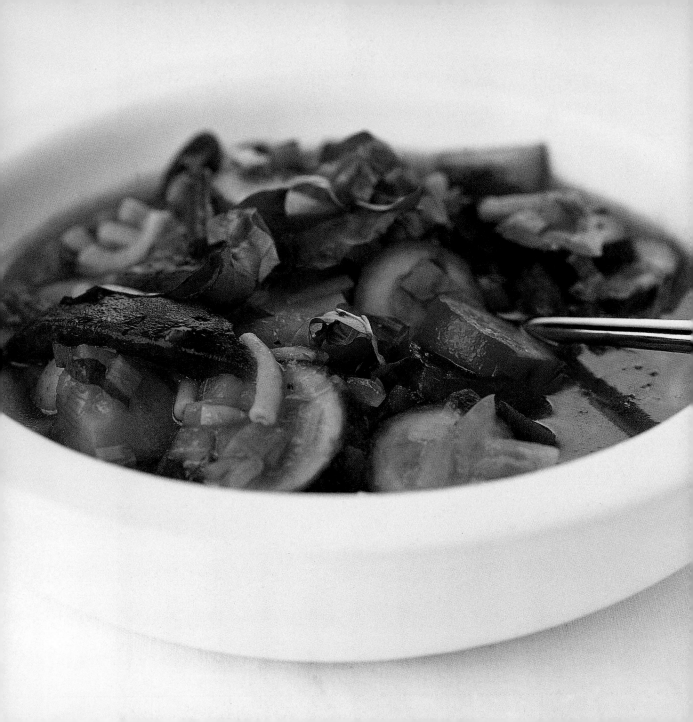

chapter four

Energy recipes

This chapter presents delicious, high-energy recipes from around the world, with many drawn from the particularly healthy diets of the East and the Mediterranean regions.

The recipes are designed to provide your body with all the nutrition

it needs throughout the day. Beginning with high-energy breakfasts,

there are also power-packed lunches and energy-sustaining dinners,

as well as juices, shakes and herbal teas which will lift your energy

and raise your spirits at any time. Now you can eat and drink healthily

all day. (Each juice recipe makes enough for one generous serving.)

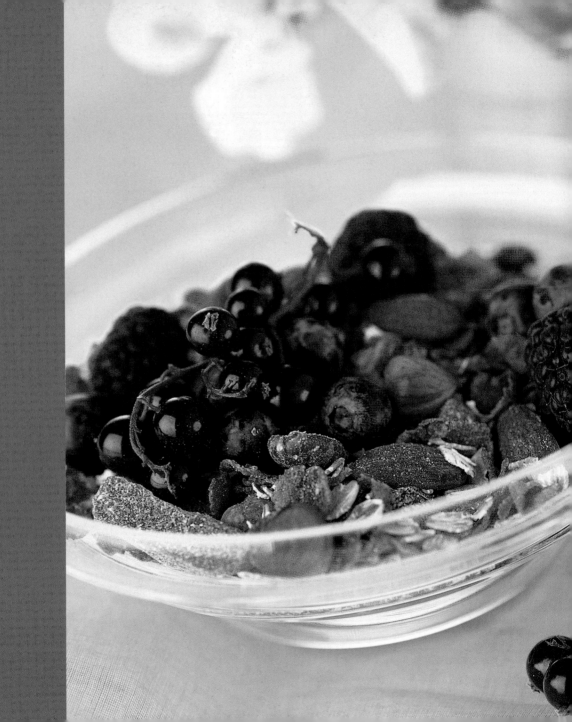

zesty**breakfasts**

kick-start the day

Muesli with fruit and nuts

Makes 1 serving

1 portion sugar-free muesli base (a mixture
of oat, wheat, barley, rice and rye)
2 tablespoons chopped nuts mixed with
seeds (e.g. walnuts, filberts, almonds,
sunflower seeds)
2 dates, chopped
2 dried apricots, chopped
1 tablespoon dried coconut
5 tablespoons seasonal fresh fruit
or berries, chopped
Soy, almond, rice or oat milk to taste

1. Mix the muesli base with the nuts, seeds,
dried fruit and coconut.
2. Sprinkle the fresh fruit or berries on top.
3. Serve with your chosen milk to taste, and
a glass of freshly squeezed grapefruit or
orange juice.

Energy boost:	✪ ✪ ✪ ✪ ✪
Nutrients:	Vitamins A, C, E & B-group; calcium, iron, magnesium, selenium, zinc; essential fatty acids
Body benefits:	Immune & digestive systems

Belgian oatmeal

Makes 1 serving

3–4 tablespoons rolled oats
1 tablespoon chopped nuts mixed with seeds
(e.g. walnuts, filberts, almonds, and
sunflower seeds)
1 tablespoon dried fruit (e.g. raisins or
apricots)
Water
Pinch of sea salt
Soy milk
$1/2$ apple, grated
Maple syrup (optional)

1. Put the oats in a saucepan with the nuts,
seeds and dried fruit.

2. Add twice the volume of water, a pinch
of sea salt and bring the mixture to a boil,
stirring continuously.
3. Simmer gently until the oats swell and
the oatmeal thickens, gradually adding a
little cold soy milk. Stir from time to time to
prevent the oatmeal sticking to the pan.
4. Serve topped with grated apple, maple
syrup and soy milk to taste.

Energy boost:	✪ ✪ ✪ ✪
Nutrients:	Vitamins E & B-group; calcium, iron, magnesium; essential fatty acids
Body benefits:	Digestive, circulatory & nervous systems; heart

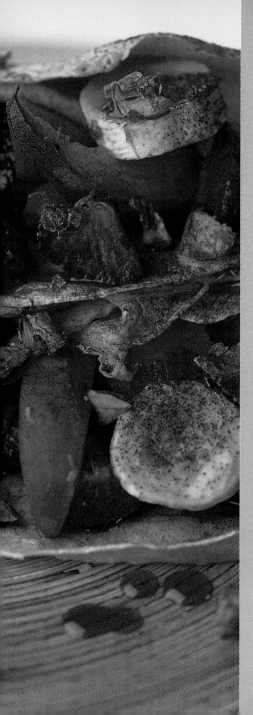

Filled pancakes

Makes 12 pancakes

Pancake batter
2 cups wheat flour
2 teaspoons baking powder
Pinch of sea salt
$^1/_2$ cup soy milk
$^2/_3$ cup water
3 tablespoons safflower oil
Grapeseed oil for cooking

1. Sift the flour and baking powder into a bowl, add salt and mix well.
2. Pour in the soy milk a little at a time, stirring continuously with a whisk.
3. Continue stirring and gradually mix in the water to form a thick batter.
4. Slowly pour in the oil and continue to stir until completely blended.
5. Allow the mixture to stand while you prepare the pancake filling.
6. Cook the pancakes one at a time in a skillet in grapeseed oil.

Pancake filling
2 bananas, thinly sliced
2 peaches, thinly sliced
2 apricots, thinly sliced
12 strawberries, chopped
Cinnamon
3 tablespoons chopped almonds or pistachios, lightly roasted in a dry skillet
Maple syrup to taste

1. Mix the bananas, peaches, apricots and strawberries in a bowl.
2. Place a couple of spoonfuls of the fruit mixture in the center of each pancake, sprinkle with cinnamon and chopped nuts, top with maple syrup and roll up. Serve immediately.

Energy boost:	✪ ✪ ✪ ✪
Nutrients:	Vitamins A, C & E; iron; essential fatty acids
Body benefit:	Immune system

Fresh fruit salad

Makes 1 serving

$^1/_2$ papaya, deseeded and sliced
1 banana, sliced
1 pear (or 1 apple), cored and sliced
1 portion fresh soft fruits or berries
    (e.g. raspberries, strawberries,
    apricots, peaches, nectarines,
    plums, cherries)
5 grapes, halved
5 tablespoons unsweetened fruit juice
1 teaspoon maple syrup (optional)

Mix together all the fruits in a bowl,
then add the fruit juice and maple
syrup. Serve with a glass of freshly
squeezed grapefrult or orange juice.

Energy boost:	✪ ✪ ✪
Nutrients:	Vitamins A & C; calcium, magnesium, zinc
Body benefits:	Immune system; detoxifying

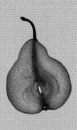

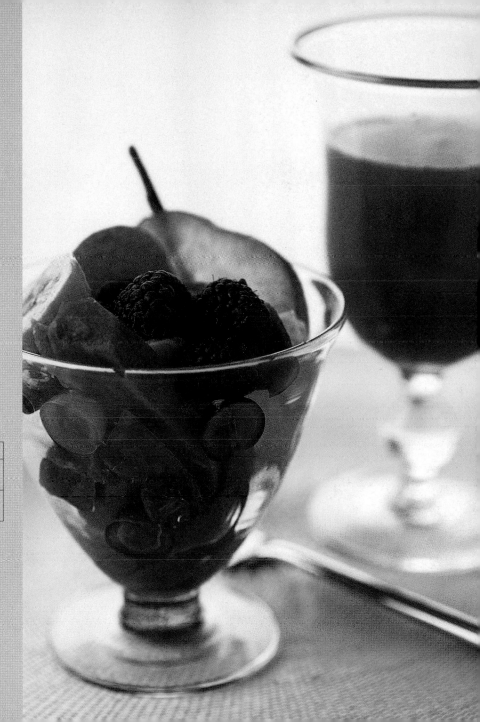

Sunrise

1 orange
1 tangerine (keep one segment aside)
1 pink grapefruit

1. Squeeze the fruit.
2. Serve together in a tall glass
garnished with a segment of tangerine.

The high vitamin C content in this juice will help
you to fight off any infections.

Energy boost:	✪ ✪ ✪
Nutrients:	Vitamins C, B$_1$ & folate; copper, magnesium, manganese, zinc
Body benefits:	Tissue-healing; nervous system; bones & muscles; blood fats

Aurore

3$\frac{1}{2}$ oz raspberries
Juice of $\frac{1}{2}$ lemon
1 tablespoon maple syrup
$\frac{1}{2}$ cup soy milk

Blend all the ingredients together
and serve.

Energy boost:	✪ ✪ ✪ ✪
Nutrients:	Vitamins C & B$_3$; calcium, magnesium, phosphorus, potassium
Body benefits:	Immune, nervous & cardiovascular systems; bones & muscles

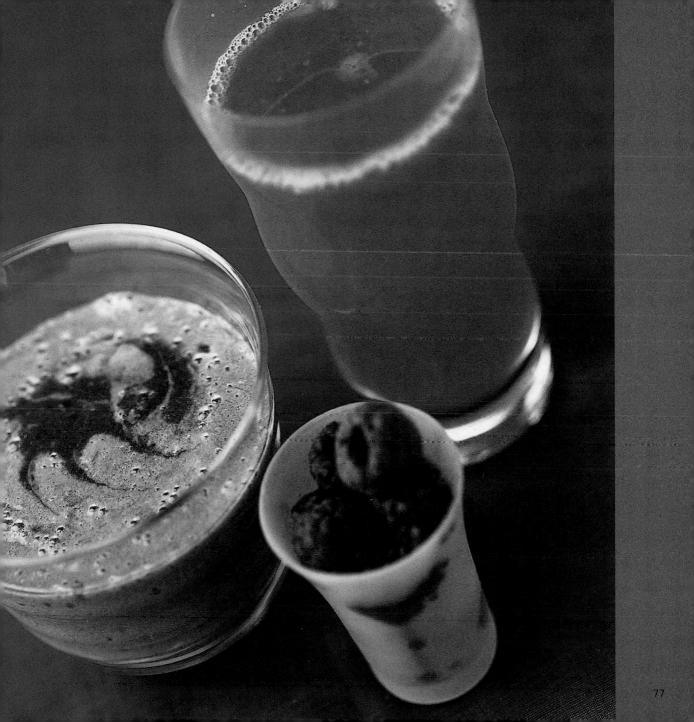

Orchard dawn

4 apples, peeled and cored
2 pears, peeled and cored
$\frac{1}{2}$ lemon, squeezed
1 teaspoon maple syrup

1. Juice the apples and pears.
2. Add the lemon juice and maple syrup.
3. Mix well and serve in a tall glass.

This is a refreshing juice that contains plenty of B-vitamins and iron, which are excellent energy boosters.

Energy boost:	✪ ✪ ✪ ✪
Nutrients:	Vitamins C, B₃ & folate; calcium, iron, magnesium, manganese
Body benefits:	Skin; mucous membranes; blood, bones & muscles; nervous system

Morning glory

1 apple, peeled and cored
1 large tomato
2 carrots
1 orange, squeezed
Slice of lemon
Sprig of mint

1. Juice the apple, tomato and carrots.
2. Add the orange juice and mix well.
3. Garnish with a slice of lemon and a sprig of mint.

Energy boost:	✪ ✪ ✪ ✪
Nutrients:	Vitamins A, C, K & B-group; calcium, copper, fluoride, iron, magnesium, manganese, zinc
Body benefits:	Antioxidant; skin & mucous membranes; blood & immune systems; eyes & nervous system

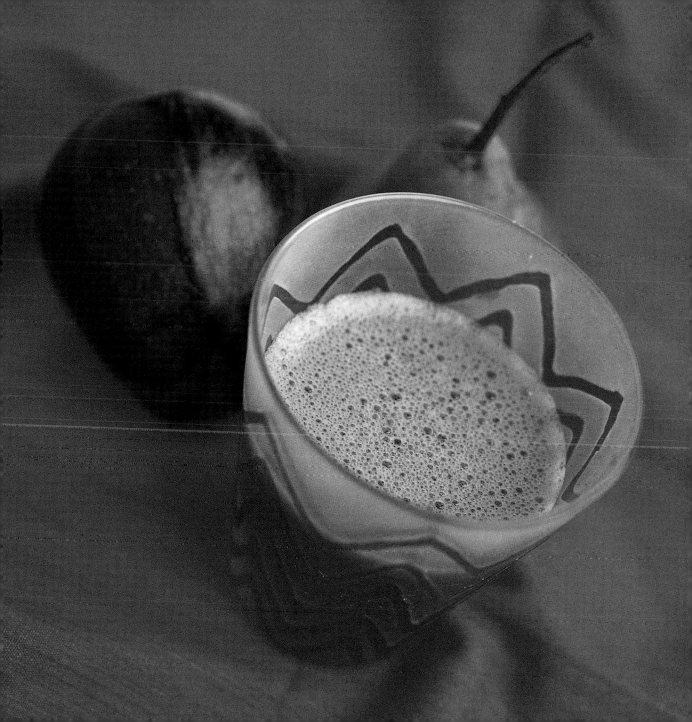

Penne pesto with Italian salad

Serves 4

Penne pesto

10 oz penne or other pasta
5 tablespoons pine nuts
1 teaspoon coarse sea salt
3 tablespoons fresh basil, finely chopped
   (or 3 teaspoons dried)
4 tablespoons extra virgin olive oil
1–2 cloves garlic, crushed

1. Boil the pasta in salted water with a little olive oil (to keep it from sticking together).
2. While the pasta is cooking, grind the pine nuts and sea salt in a mortar or blender.
3. Add the basil, olive oil and garlic to the ground pine nuts and salt, and mix well.
4. Transfer the pesto to a small bowl.
5. Put the cooked pasta in a separate dish. Serve the pesto and pasta with Italian salad.

Italian salad

1 small radicchio, shredded
1 cup fresh peas, shelled
1 carrot, finely diced
2 ripe tomatoes, diced
1 yellow pepper, diced
$1/2$ bulb of fennel, diced
$1/2$ red onion, diced
4 radishes, sliced
4 button mushrooms, thinly sliced
Fresh basil leaves to garnish

Put the shredded radicchio in a large salad bowl and add the rest of the ingredients in the order shown above. Garnish with basil and serve with walnut dressing.

Walnut dressing

Juice of $1/2$ a ripe lemon
Sea salt and black pepper
1 teaspoon soy sauce
2 teaspoons maple syrup
1 teaspoon Dijon mustard
$1/2$ teaspoon curry powder
1 teaspoon tahini
$2/3$ cup walnut oil
Extra virgin olive oil to taste

1. Put the lemon juice, salt, pepper, soy sauce, maple syrup, mustard and curry powder into a bowl and whisk with a fork.
2. Add the tahini and continue whisking until the consistency is smooth.
3. Gradually stir in the walnut oil.
4. Add olive oil to taste.

Energy boost:	✪ ✪ ✪ ✪ ✪
Nutrients:	Vitamins A, C, E, niacin, thiamin & folate; calcium, iron, magnesium, manganese, zinc; essential fatty acids
Body benefits:	Heart; circulatory system

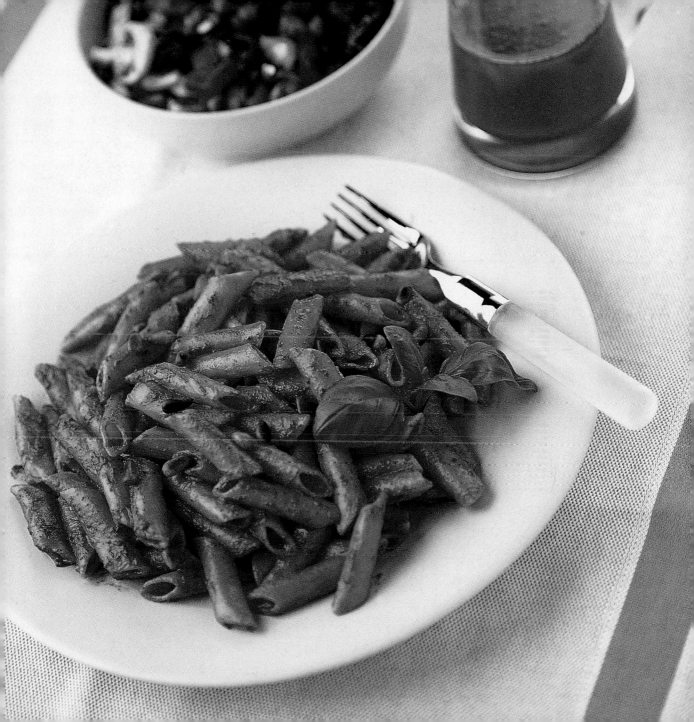

Baba ganoush
with three-root salad

Serves 4

Baba ganoush
1 medium eggplant
1 clove garlic, crushed
3 tablespoons tahini
3 tablespoons lemon juice
Sea salt
Fresh parsley, finely chopped, to garnish

1. Prick the eggplant with a fork, then place under
a moderate grill, turning frequently until the skin is
charred and loosened from the flesh.
2. Cool the eggplant by holding it under running water for
a minute, then cut in half lengthwise and scrape out the
flesh with a tablespoon.
3. Chop the flesh finely, put it in a bowl and mix with the
garlic, tahini, lemon juice and salt.
4. Put in a serving bowl, garnish with parsley and serve.

Three-root salad
3-4 medium carrots, scrubbed
1 small beet, peeled
$^1/_4$ medium celeriac, peeled

Grate all the ingredients, mix together in a salad bowl and
serve with pita bread and baba ganoush.

Energy boost:	✪ ✪ ✪
Nutrients:	Vitamins A, C, E & folate; calcium, iron, zinc
Body benefit:	Immune system

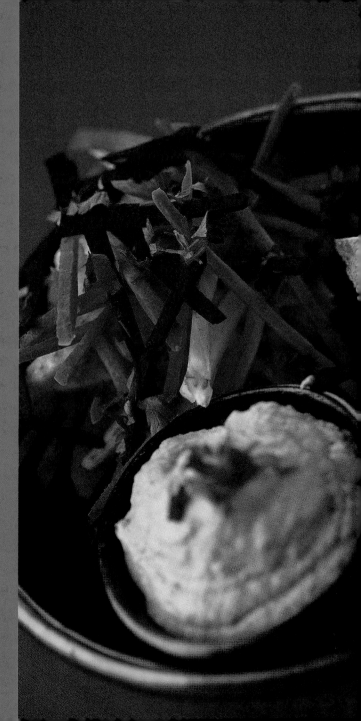

Tabouleh Orientale
with Korean cucumber

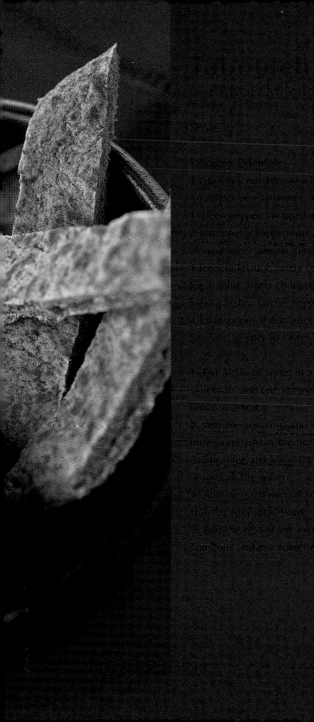

Serves 4

Tabouleh Orientale
1 cup couscous (dry weight)
4 tablespoons safflower oil
1 green pepper, chopped into small cubes
2 tomatoes, chopped into small cubes
4 small green onions, finely sliced
1 iceberg lettuce, finely chopped
Fresh mint, finely chopped
Fresh parsley, finely chopped
4 tablespoons lemon juice
Sea salt, pepper to taste

1. Put 1 cup of water in a medium-sized
saucepan, add one teaspoon of salt, and
bring to a boil.
2. Add the couscous and remove the pan
immediately from the heat.
3. Stir once, and allow the couscous to
absorb all the water.
4. Add the safflower oil to the couscous and
transfer to a salad bowl.
5. Add the rest of the ingredients to the
couscous and mix together.

Korean cucumber
1 medium cucumber, finely sliced
1 medium onion, finely sliced
2 teaspoons sea salt
4 tablespoons lemon juice
Pinch of cayenne pepper
2 tablespoons tahini
1 tablespoon sesame oil

1. Put the cucumber and onion slices in
a bowl.
2. Sprinkle over the salt and mix well.
3. Add the lemon juice, cayenne pepper,
tahini and sesame oil.
4. Mix again, and serve with tabouleh
Orientale.

Energy boost:	✪ ✪ ✪
Nutrients:	Vitamins C, E & B-group, calcium, iron, zinc, essential fatty acids
Body benefits:	Immune system

Amanida Catalana

Serves 4

1 Little Gem lettuce, shredded
$^1/_2$ yellow pepper, cut in long thin slices
$^1/_2$ red pepper, cut in long thin slices
2 tomatoes, cut in thin boats
2 tablespoons corn
1 red onion, finely sliced
2 tablespoons capers
2 tablespoons brazil nuts, finely chopped

1. Place the shredded lettuce on a flat salad plate and add the yellow and red peppers to form stripes on the lettuce.
2. Decorate with the tomatoes and corn.
3. Garnish with the onion, capers and brazil nuts. Serve with rice and walnut dressing (see p.80).

Energy boost:	✪ ✪ ✪ ✪
Nutrients:	Vitamins A, C & B-group; calcium, iron, magnesium, selenium, zinc; essential fatty acids,
Body benefits:	Immune, circulatory, digestive & nervous systems

Soupe au pistou

3 tablespoons extra virgin olive oil
1 leek, sliced
2 onions, halved and sliced lengthwise
2–3 cloves garlic, crushed
$^1/_4$ medium celeriac, diced
2 carrots, chopped
2 medium potatoes, diced
3 tomatoes, peeled and cut into thin boats
1 generous cup green beans, sliced
1 zucchini, chopped
3 pints vegetable stock or water
$1^1/_2$ cups cooked navy beans
3 tablespoons fresh basil (or 3 teaspoons dried) finely chopped
2 oz small macaroni
Sea salt and pepper

1. Heat the oil in a large pan and soften (but do not brown) the leek, onions and garlic.
2. Add the celeriac, carrots and potatoes, stirring continously as they heat through, then put in the tomatoes.
3. Cook for 2 minutes. Add the green beans and zucchini.
4. Pour in the stock, bring to a boil, and simmer. Add the navy beans and 2 tablespoons of fresh basil. Boil again.
5. Add the macaroni, salt and pepper. Simmer for a further 10–15 minutes. Add the rest of the basil, adjust seasoning and serve with thick slices of fresh bread.

Energy boost:	✪ ✪ ✪ ✪
Nutrients:	Vitamins A, C, E, thiamin, niacin & folate; calcium, iron, magnesium, manganese, zinc
Body benefits:	Heart; circulatory, nervous & urino-genital systems; skin

Gazpacho de Campo

Serves 4

1 cucumber, finely chopped
8 medium tomatoes, peeled and
  finely chopped
1 onion, finely chopped
1 green pepper, finely chopped
2 cloves garlic, finely chopped
5 tablespoons extra virgin olive oil
3 tablespoons lemon juice
3 tablespoons raspberry vinegar
Sea salt and pepper
1 small bunch fresh dill, finely chopped
Croutons and ice cubes

1. Set aside a quarter of each of the chopped vegetables, except the garlic, and blend the rest with the olive oil, lemon juice and vinegar to a thick, smooth consistency.
2. Season to taste, transfer to a soup tureen, and chill for at least an hour.
3. Garnish with dill and serve with rest of finely chopped vegetables, croutons and ice cubes in separate side dishes.

Energy boost:	✪ ✪ ✪
Nutrients:	Vitamins A, E, B$_6$ & niacin; iron, zinc; essential fatty acids
Body benefits:	Immune, circulatory & urino-genital systems; skin

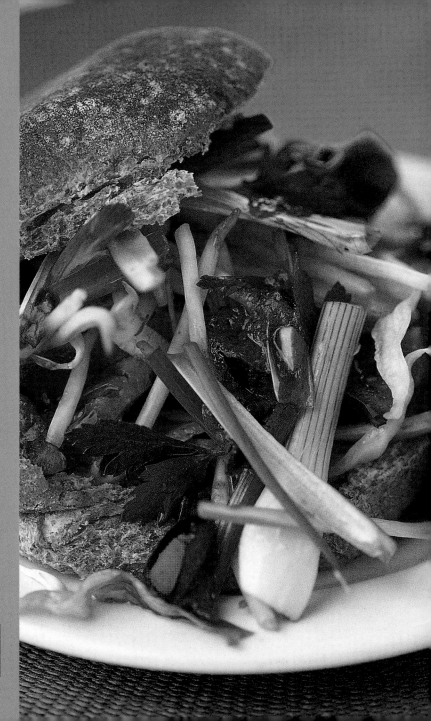

Crunchy Spanish salad
with hot sesame sauce

Serves 4

Crunchy Spanish salad
1 small Iceberg lettuce, finely shredded
1 small green pepper, finely chopped
2 stalks celery, finely chopped
1 carrot, grated
1 handful grapes, halved and seeded
1 handful bean sprouts

Put the lettuce in a large bowl with the pepper, celery and carrot. Garnish with the grapes and bean sprouts.

Hot sesame sauce
3 tablespoons tahini
3 tablespoons water
3 tablespoons lemon juice
1 clove garlic, crushed
1 teaspoon fresh ginger, grated
Pinch of cayenne pepper
$^{1}/_{4}$ teaspoon sea salt

Mix all the ingredients well and heat gently in a saucepan. Serve with crunchy Spanish salad and thick slices of crusty bread.

Energy boost:	✪ ✪ ✪
Nutrients:	Vitamins A, C & folate; zinc
Body benefits:	Immune system

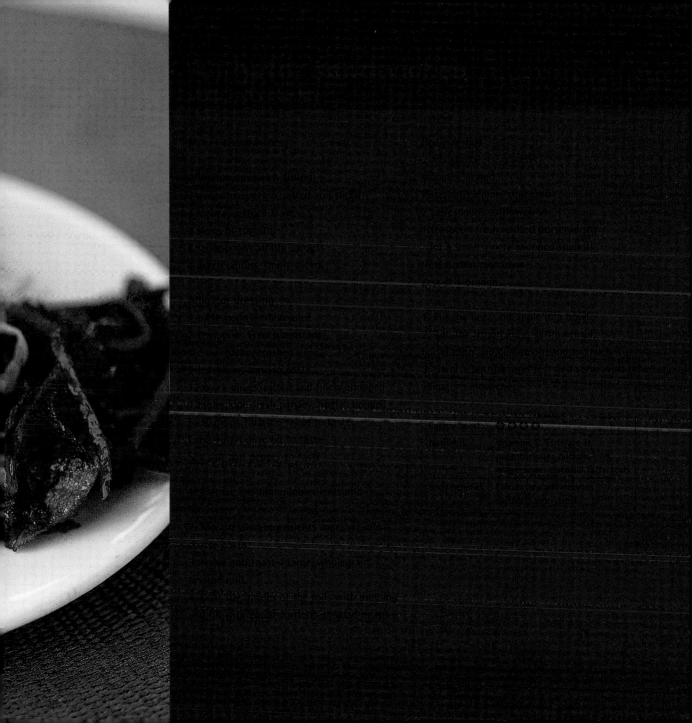

Sunflower pâté
with tropicana salad

Serves 4

Sunflower pâté
1 cup sunflower seeds
1 tablespoon soy sauce
2 tablespoons extra virgin olive oil
1 shallot, finely chopped
1¹/₂ cups cooked green lentils
1–2 tablespoons lemon juice
1 teaspoon ground coriander
¹/₂ teaspoon black pepper
Salt to taste

1. "Toast" the sunflower seeds in a dry skillet.
2. When they begin to pop and brown, turn off the heat and add the soy sauce.
3. Stir well, then put in a mortar or food processor and grind to a coarse powder.
4. Put the oil in the skillet, add the chopped shallot and soften for a few minutes over a low heat.
5. Put the ground sunflower seeds and cooked shallot in a food processor with the other ingredients and blend to a smooth consistency.
6. Serve with fresh French bread and tropicana salad.

Tropicana salad
4 slices fresh pineapple, peeled and diced
1 papaya, peeled and diced
¹/₂ green pepper, finely chopped
1 banana, finely chopped
1 handful raisins

2 tablespoons freshly grated (or dried) coconut
1 teaspoon fresh ginger, grated
4 crisp Iceberg lettuce leaves
4 lychees, peeled, pitted and halved
   to garnish (optional)

Tropicana dressing
²/₃ cup coconut milk
¹/₂ teaspoon curry powder
1 teaspoon mustard
2 teaspoons lemon juice
2 teaspoons maple syrup
Pinch of sea salt

1. Mix the pineapple, papaya, green pepper, banana, raisins, coconut and grated ginger in a bowl.
2. Place an equal amount on each lettuce leaf.
3. Arrange the leaves on a serving plate.
4. Mix all the tropicana dressing ingredients and add a teaspoonful to each leaf. Garnish with lychees.

Energy boost:	✪ ✪ ✪ ✪ ✪
Nutrients:	Vitamins C, E & niacin; calcium, iron, magnesium, manganese, zinc
Body benefits:	Immune, circulatory, nervous & urino-genital systems; bones

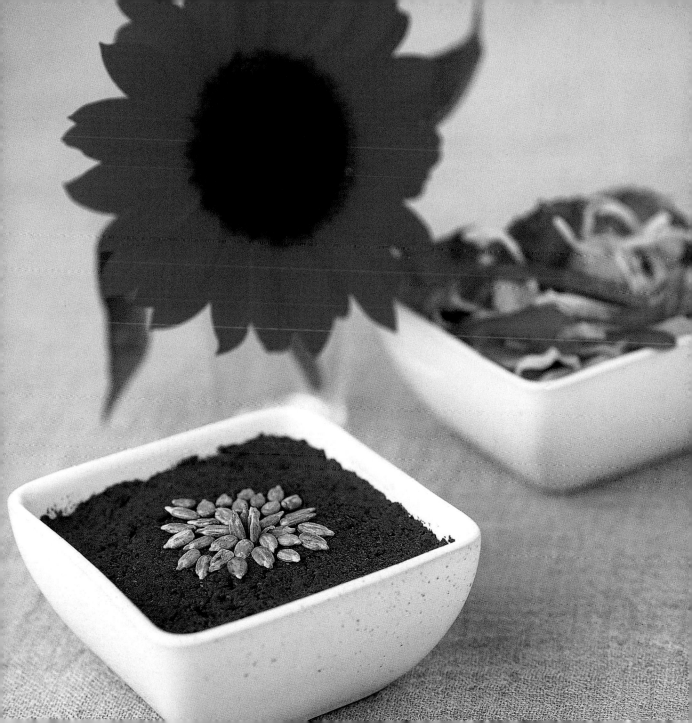

Spicy garbanzo beans

Serves 4

2 tablespoons extra virgin olive oil
1 teaspoon ground cumin
1 teaspoon ground coriander seeds
2 cloves garlic, finely chopped
1 onion, chopped
2¹/₂ cups cooked garbanzo beans
6 tomatoes, peeled and chopped
2 tablespoons fresh parsley, finely chopped
1 teaspoon dried thyme
Pinch of chile pepper
1 teaspoon fresh, grated ginger
¹/₃ cup water or vegetable stock
Sea salt and pepper

1. Heat the oil gently in a large saucepan or wok.
2. Add the cumin, coriander seeds, garlic and onion.
3. Stir-fry for 3–4 minutes, add the garbanzo beans, and then
the rest of the ingredients.
4. Bring to a boil and simmer gently for 15 minutes, adding a
little water from time to time if necessary.
5. Adjust seasoning and serve with lightly steamed, fresh,
green beans, and basmati rice cooked with red lentils
(known as khichuri).

Energy boost:	✪ ✪ ✪ ✪ ✪	
Nutrients:	Vitamins C, E & B-group; calcium, iron, magnesium, zinc	
Body benefit:	Whole body	

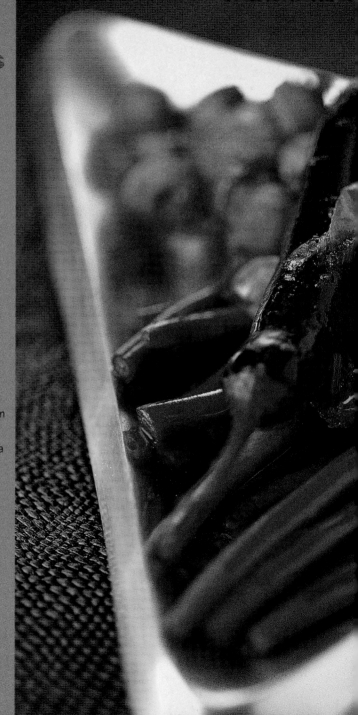

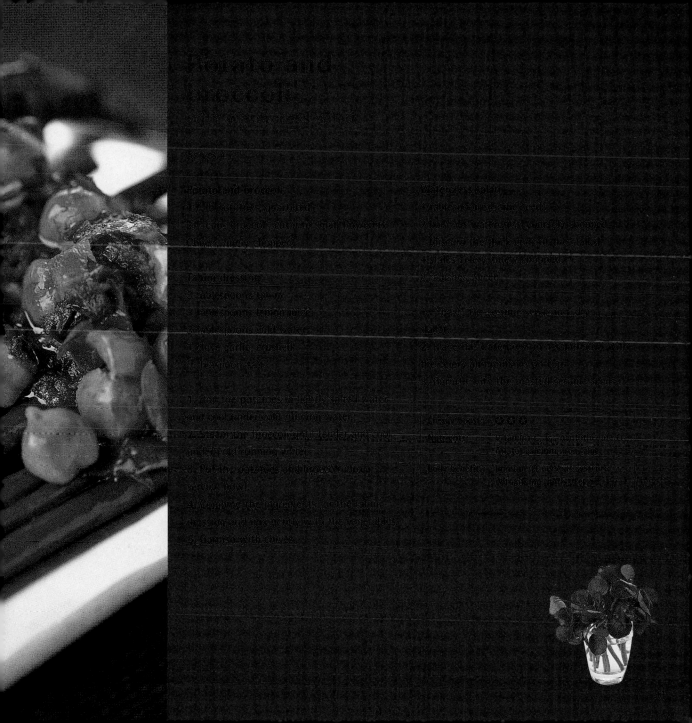

Potato and
broccoli

with watercress salad

Serves 4

Potato and broccoli
4 potatoes, quartered
2 heads broccoli, cut into small flowerets
1 onion, finely chopped

Tahini dressing
3 tablespoons tahini
3 tablespoons lemon juice
3 tablespoons cold water
1 clove garlic, crushed
½ teaspoon salt

1. Boil the potatoes in lightly salted water
and cool under cold running water.
2. Steam the broccoli until tender and cool
under cold running water.
3. Put the potatoes and broccoli into a
serving bowl.
4. Combine the ingredients for the tahini
dressing and mix gently with the vegetables.
5. Garnish with parsley.

Watercress salad
1 cup pomegranate seeds
2 bunches watercress, coarsely chopped
(remove the thick stems of the stalks)
4 stalks celery, finely chopped
4 parsley, chopped

1. Mash the sesame seeds into a dry
skillet.
2. Place the watercress, pomegranate and
the celery and mix well in a bowl.
3. Garnish with the toasted sesame seeds.

Energy boost
Nutrients   vitamins C, E, and potassium
             folic acid and magnesium
Body benefits detoxifies, improves digestion
             blood sugar balance

Strawberry shake

10 strawberries, stalks removed
1 tablespoon natural soy yogurt
1 teaspoon honey (or 1 tablespoon
   maple syrup)
Pinch of vanilla powder
1 sprig fresh mint

Energy boost:	✪ ✪ ✪
Nutrients:	Vitamins C, K & pantothenate; calcium, magnesium, potassium
Body benefits:	Tissue-healing; immune & nervous systems; blood, bones & muscles

1. Blend all the ingredients for about 30 seconds.
2. Serve garnished with a sprig of mint.

Tropical shake

$^1/_2$ guava, peeled and pitted
$^1/_2$ pineapple, peeled
$^1/_2$ mango, peeled and pitted
2 lychees, peeled and pitted
1 slice of lime

Energy boost:	✪ ✪ ✪ ✪ ✪
Nutrients:	Vitamins A & C; copper
Body benefits:	Immune & nervous systems; skin; eyes; blood fats; bones

1. Juice the fruits.
2. Serve in a tall glass decorated
with a slice of lime.
3. Drink through a thick straw.

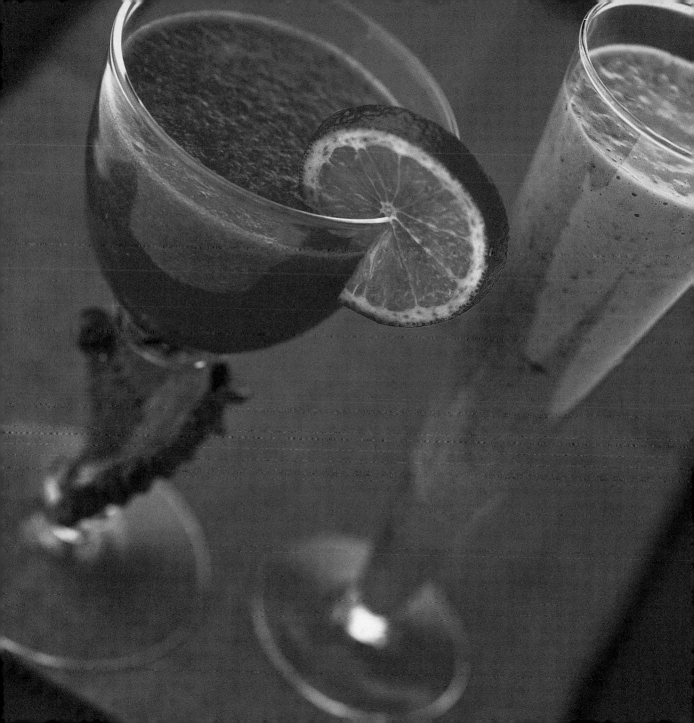

Bananarama

1 banana, peeled
1 chunk fresh coconut (or 1 teaspoon shredded)
$^1/_2$ cup soy milk
1 teaspoon honey

1. Blend all the ingredients together for about
30 seconds.
2. Serve chilled.

Bananas are excellent for providing an instant burst of energy. Drink
this filling shake at any time of the day.

Energy boost:	✪ ✪ ✪ ✪
Nutrients:	Vitamins B$_3$, biotin & B$_6$; calcium, magnesium, manganese, phosphorus, potassium
Body benefits:	Skin & hair; bones & muscles; nervous, cardiovascular & immune systems

Apricot lassi

4 fresh apricots, peeled and pitted
1 banana, peeled
$^1/_4$ cup almond milk
1 pinch of cinnamon

1. Blend the apricots and banana with the almond milk.
2. Serve garnished with a pinch of cinnamon.

A lassi is a traditional drink in India, where it is known for its cooling,
refreshing properties.

Energy boost:	✪ ✪ ✪ ✪ ✪
Nutrients:	Vitamins E, B$_2$, B$_3$, B$_6$ & biotin; cobalt, fluoride, iron, magnesium, manganese, potassium
Body benefits:	Immune, nervous & cardiovascular systems; bones & muscles; teeth

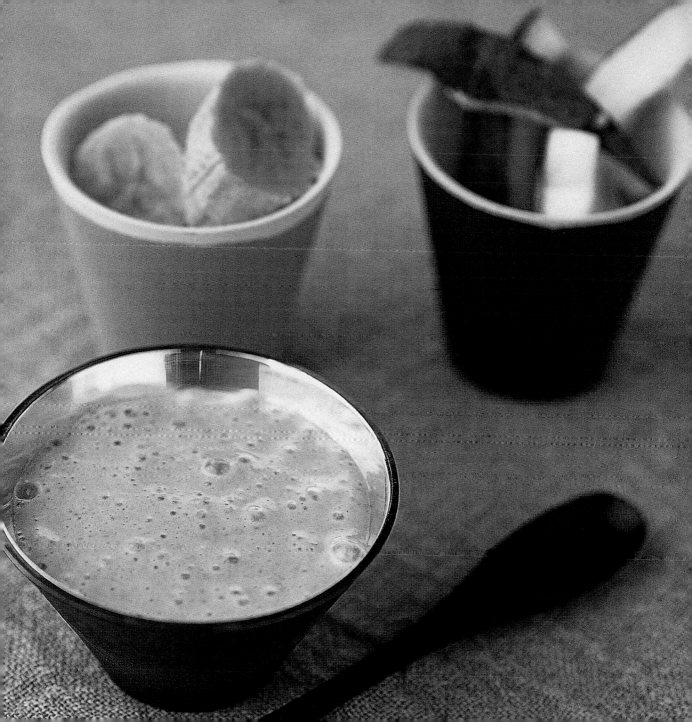

Peach pleaser

2 fresh peaches, peeled and pitted
2 fresh apricots, peeled and pitted
$^1/_4$ cup soy milk
1 tablespoon maple syrup
1 pinch vanilla powder

Blend all the ingredients together and serve.

Energy boost:	✪ ✪ ✪ ✪
Nutrients:	Vitamins C & B$_3$; calcium, cobalt, fluoride, iron, magnesium, phosphorus, potassium, zinc
Body benefits:	Immune & cardiovascular systems; skin; bones & teeth; tissue-healing

Ace

9 oz carrots
1 orange, squeezed
$^1/_2$ lemon, squeezed

1. Juice the carrots.
2. Add the orange and lemon juice, mix well and serve.

This juice is packed with antioxidants to help the body fight infection.

Energy boost:	✪ ✪ ✪ ✪
Nutrients:	Vitamins A, K, C, B$_1$, B$_3$, B$_6$ & folate; calcium, copper, iron, magnesium, manganese, phosphorus, zinc
Body benefits:	Immune, cardiovascular & nervous systems; blood & bones; skin; tissue-healing

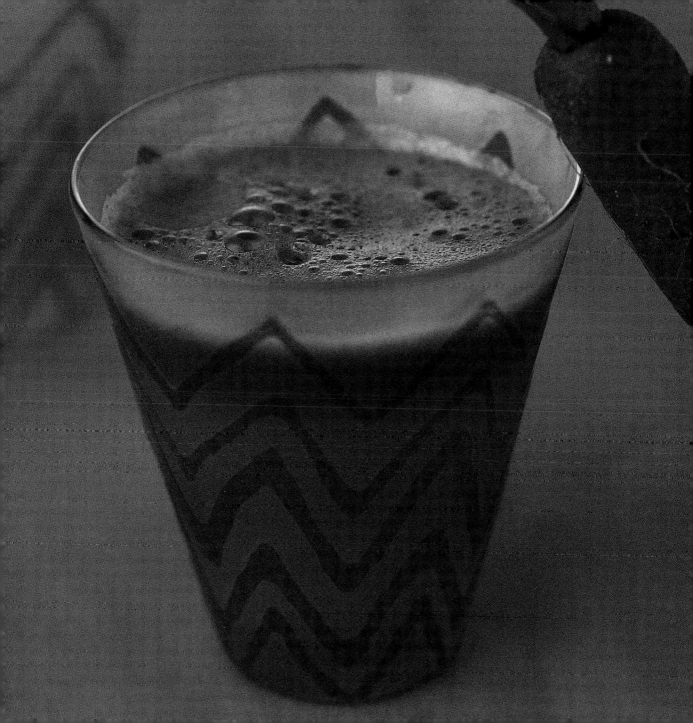

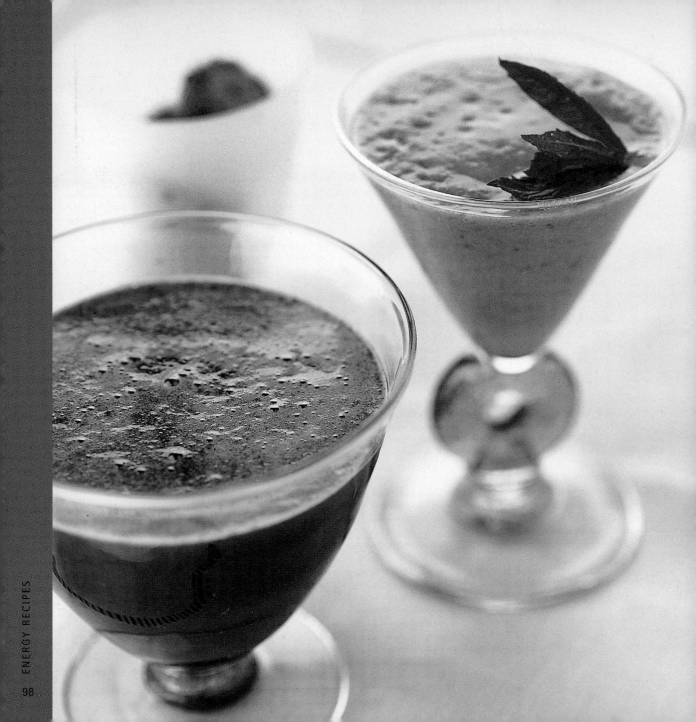

Ruby reviver

1 tomato
1 stalk celery
$1/4$ lemon, peeled
$1/4$ cucumber, peeled
$1/2$ beet, peeled
2 carrots
1–2 sprigs of fresh lovage (or basil, chives or parsley)
Sea salt and black pepper to taste
1–2 drops Tabasco sauce (optional)
Slice of lemon to garnish

1. Cut the ingredients into chunks and press them through the juicer, one at a time.
2. Add sea salt and black pepper to taste and pour into a tall glass with one or two drops of Tabasco sauce.
3. Decorate glass with a slice of lemon and drink through a thick straw.

Energy boost:	✪ ✪ ✪
Nutrients:	Vitamins A, C, folate & pantothenate; all minerals
Body benefits:	Nervous & immune systems; detoxifying

Strawberry and banana smoothie

$2/3$ cup thick apple juice
8 fresh strawberries, stalks removed
1 banana, peeled
Sprig of fresh mint

Energy boost:	✪ ✪ ✪
Nutrient:	Vitamin C
Body benefit:	Immune system

Put the apple juice, strawberries and banana in a blender and blend for 30 seconds. Serve in a tall glass, garnished with fresh mint.

Crispy lettuce rolls
with almand dressing

Makes 12 rolls

Crispy lettuce rolls
2 green onions, finely chopped
1 avocado, peeled, pitted and diced
1 carrot, grated
1 stalk celery, finely chopped
$^{1}/_{2}$ red pepper, deseeded and finely chopped

1 handful of fresh sprouts (sunflower, alfalfa or bean)
12 large lettuce leaves (a mixture of green and red)
A few edible flowers (e.g. nasturtium, marigold or borage), or some sprigs of fresh herbs (e.g. basil, parsley or cilantro)

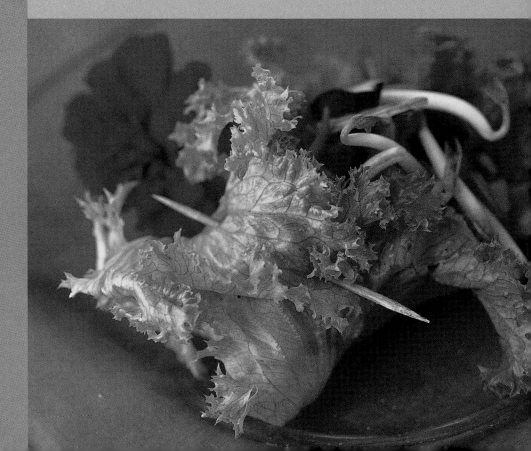

1. Combine the green onions, avocado, carrot, celery, red pepper and sprouts in a bowl, and mix well.
2. Place a tablespoon of the mixture in the middle of a lettuce leaf and add a spoonful of almond dressing.
3. Fold the two sides of the leaf into the middle, then roll it up from stalk to tip, and fasten with a toothpick.
4. Repeat with the other leaves.
5. Serve garnished with edible flowers or herb sprigs.

Almond dressing

4 tablespoons almond butter
4 tablespoons lemon juice
4 tablespoons water
Sea salt and pepper to taste

1. Stir together almond butter, lemon juice and water.
2. Season with salt and black pepper.

For variety, try the following variation:
6 tablespoons extra virgin olive oil
1 clove garlic, crushed
2 tablespoons almond butter
4 or 5 fresh tarragon leaves, finely chopped
   (or $^1/_2$ teaspoon dried)
4 tablespoons lemon juice; sea salt and pepper to taste

1. Place all ingredients in a bowl and mix well.
2. Season with salt and black pepper.

Energy boost:	✪ ✪ ✪ ✪ ✪	
Nutrients:	Vitamins A, C, E & B-group; calcium, iron, magnesium, zinc; essential fatty acids	
Body benefits:	Nervous, circulatory & immune systems; anti-stress	

Greek olive and lime pâté

15 Greek olives, pitted and finely chopped
1 cup cooked butter beans
Juice of $^1/_2$ lime
1 tablespoon extra virgin olive oil
Small pinch of cayenne pepper
Sea salt and pepper to taste
Slices of lime and radish to garnish

1. Combine all the ingredients in a mixing bowl and mash to a smooth consistency.
2. Transfer to serving dish and garnish with thin slices of lime and crisp red radish.
3. Serve with rough oatcakes or melba toast.

Energy boost:	✪ ✪ ✪ ✪	
Nutrients:	Vitamins C, E, niacin, folate, & pantothenate; calcium, iron, magnesium, zinc; essential fatty acids	
Body benefits:	Nervous & immune systems; bones; anti-stress	

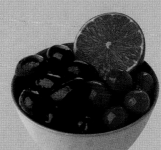

Pistachio and raisin halva

1 cup toasted sesame seeds
2 tablespoons raw sugar
2 tablespoons unsalted pistachio nuts, finely chopped
1 tablespoon raisins
2 tablespoons honey

Energy boost:	✪ ✪ ✪ ✪
Nutrients:	Vitamins E, niacin, biotin, & pantothenate; calcium, iron, magnesium, selenium, zinc
Body benefits:	Immune, nervous and endocrine systems; skin & hair; anti-stress

1. Toast the sesame seeds in a dry pan, allow to cool, then grind with the sugar in a mortar to a powder.
2. Put in a bowl, add the rest of the ingredients and knead to form a stiff batter.
3. Shape the batter into a rectangular loaf.
4. Refrigerate for half an hour before slicing and serving.

For variety, try using other nuts in place of pistachios.

Mint and raisin spread

1³/₄ cups raisins
A handful of fresh mint leaves
Hot water

Energy boost:	✪ ✪ ✪
Nutrients:	Vitamins C, niacin, biotin & pantothenate; iron
Body benefits:	Immune, circulatory & digestive systems; skin & hair; anti-stress

1. Put the raisins and the mint in a blender, adding a little hot water at a time until the mixture blends to form a smooth paste.
2. Serve spread on freshly toasted, wholegrain muffins.

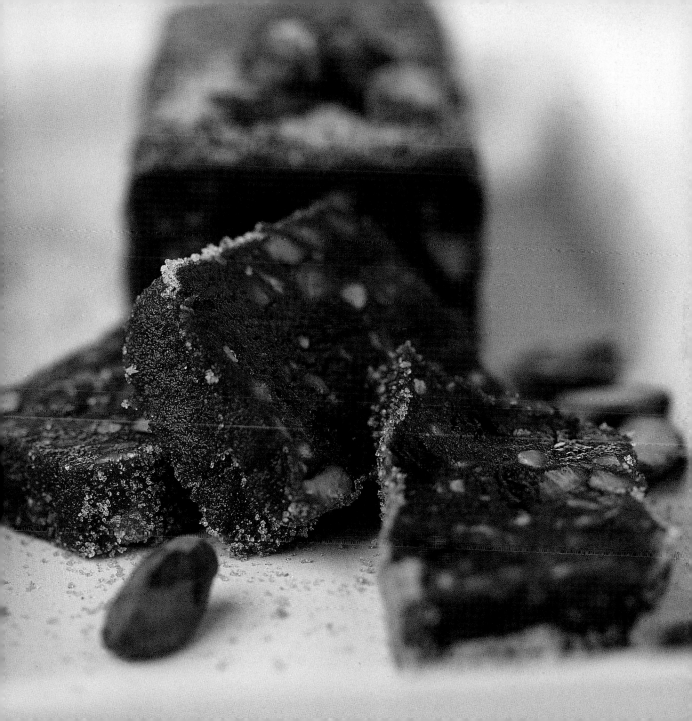

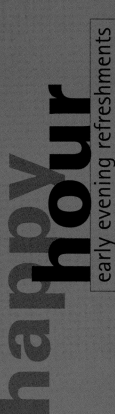

Glamorgan glee

1 cup peppermint tea
$1/2$ teaspoon lemon zest
1 pinch cinnamon
1 whole clove
$1/2$ teaspoon fresh grated ginger
1 teaspoon maple syrup
1 orange, squeezed
Fizzy water and ice cubes to taste
Fresh mint and slice of lemon

1. Make the peppermint tea.
2. While it infuses, place the lemon zest, cinnamon, clove and ginger in a bowl.
3. Add the maple syrup, orange juice and brewed peppermint tea.
4. Leave to cool.
5. Just before serving, add fizzy water and ice cubes.
6. Garnish with fresh mint and a slice of lemon.

Energy boost:	✪ ✪ ✪
Nutrients:	Vitamins C, B$_6$ & folate; copper, magnesium, manganese
Body benefits:	Immune, digestive, nervous & cardiovascular systems

Starburst

$1/2$ cup water
1 teaspoon honey
1–2 whole cloves
1 teaspoon fresh grated ginger
1 pinch cinnamon
1 piece star anise
1 orange, peeled
2 thick pineapple slices, peeled
1 slice of lime
Ice cubes

1. Pour the water into a small saucepan. Add the honey and spices.

2. Bring to a boil, turn the heat down and simmer, stirring occasionally, until the liquid reduces by half. Strain and leave to cool.
3. Juice the orange and pineapple. Mix with the cooled liquid.
4. Serve with the lime and ice cubes.

Energy boost:	✪ ✪ ✪ ✪
Nutrients:	Vitamins C, B$_6$ & folate; copper, magnesium, manganese, zinc
Body benefits:	Immune & nervous systems; blood, skin & bones; tissue-healing

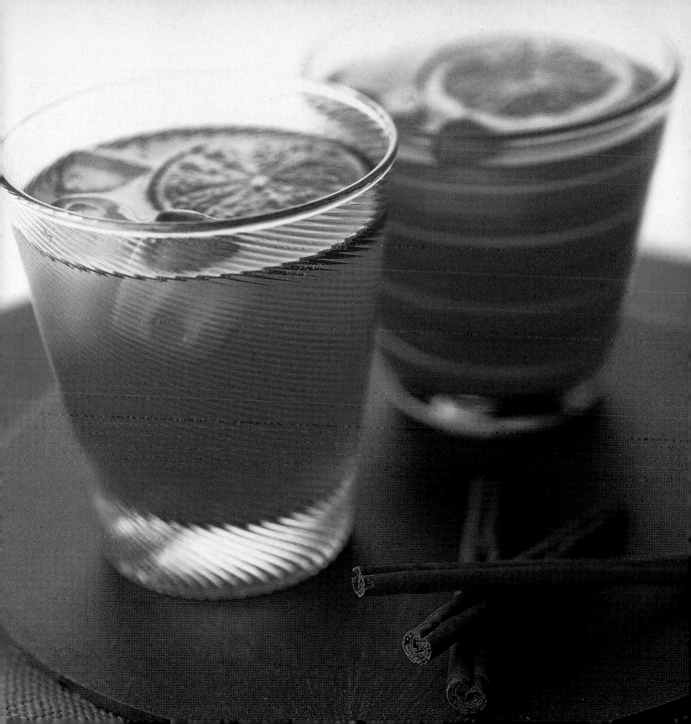

Apple fizz

4 eating apples, peeled and cored
$\frac{1}{2}$ lemon, squeezed
$\frac{1}{2}$ cup fizzy water
Ice cubes

1. Juice the apples.
2. Add the lemon juice.
3. Pour into a serving glass, add fizzy water and ice
cubes and serve.

Research shows that regularly eating apples improves breathing
by increasing lung capacity.

Energy boost:	✪ ✪ ✪ ✪ ✪
Nutrients:	Vitamins C, B_3 & folate; calcium, iron, magnesium
Body benefits:	Immune, nervous & cardiovascular systems; bones

Lemon spring

Juice of a lemon
1 tablespoon honey
Still or fizzy water to taste
1 sprig lemon balm
Ice cubes

1. Pour the lemon juice into a glass.
2. Add the honey to the lemon juice and mix well.
3. Dilute with the water, add ice cubes, and serve with a floating
sprig of lemon balm.

When lemon juice was added to sailors' rations in 1772 scurvy
vanished from the British Navy within two years.

Energy boost:	✪ ✪ ✪ ✪
Nutrients:	Vitamins C & B_3; calcium
Body benefits:	Immune system; skin; bones

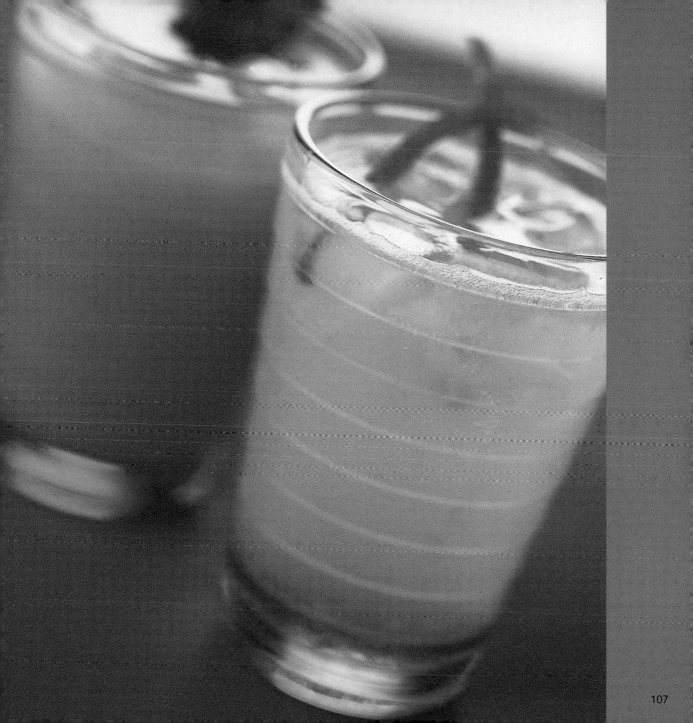

Elderflower "champagne"

The creamy-white blossoms of the graceful elder herald the beginning of summer, and have a long history of medicinal use by traditional herbalists. They are considered to have "hot and dry" properties, making them excellent protectors against colds and 'flu and useful in easing chronic conditions such as arthritis. They also help the body to detoxify by improving circulation and encouraging perspiration. Fragrant and relaxing, elderflower champagne is a delicious way to promote good health.

1 head of fresh elderflowers
1 thick slice of lemon
2 teaspoons maple syrup
½ cup boiling water
Fizzy water to taste

1. Place the elderflowers in a small bowl and pour the boiling water over.
2. Add the lemon slice and maple syrup.
3. Cover and leave to cool.
4. Strain and dilute 50/50 with chilled fizzy water just before serving.

Energy boost:	✪ ✪ ✪ ✪
Nutrient:	Vitamin C
Body benefit:	Upper respiratory system

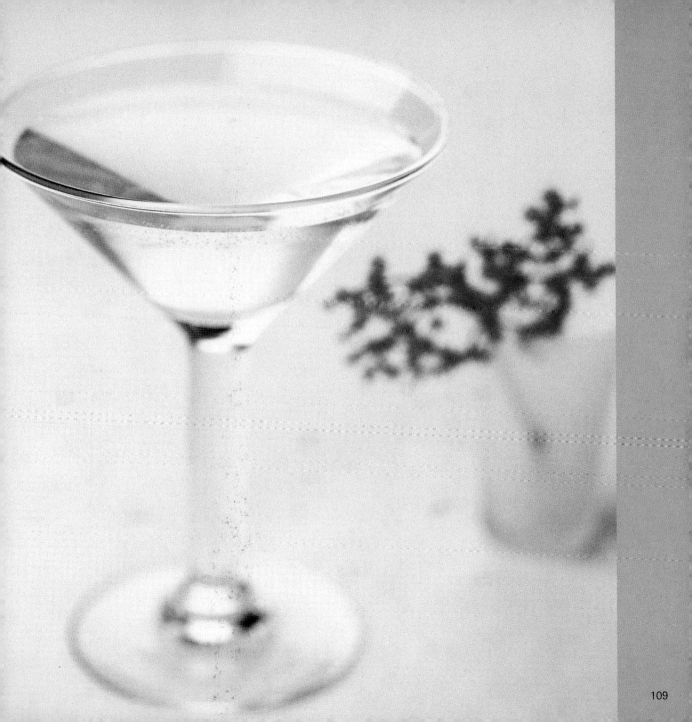

G&T

1 ruby-red grapefruit
$1/2$ cup Indian tonic water
1 slice of lemon

1. Juice the grapefruit and pour into
a tall glass.
2. Add tonic water.
3. Garnish with a slice of lemon.
4. Serve with plenty of ice.

Energy boost:	✪ ✪ ✪
Nutrient:	Vitamin C
Body benefits:	Immune system; blood fats

Melon magic

$1/4$ water melon
$1/4$ cantaloupe melon
$1/4$ honeydew melon
1 pinch of cinnamon

1. Peel and seed the melons.
2. Blend together. Serve poured over
ice cubes in a tall glass.
3. Garnish with a sprinkle of cinnamon.

Energy boost:	✪ ✪ ✪ ✪
Nutrients:	Vitamin A; copper
Body benefits:	Skin; immune & nervous systems; blood & bones

Tim's toms

2 large fresh tomatoes
1 teaspoon tamari
1 pinch fresh thyme
Salt, pepper and Tabasco to taste
1 slice of lemon

1. Juice the tomatoes.
2. Stir in the tamari, thyme, salt, pepper and
Tabasco.
3. Pour into a glass and float the slice of
lemon on top.

Energy boost:	✪ ✪ ✪
Nutrients:	Vitamins A, B_3, pantothenate & B_6; fluoride, zinc
Body benefits:	Immune & nervous systems; skin; bones; teeth; tissue–healing

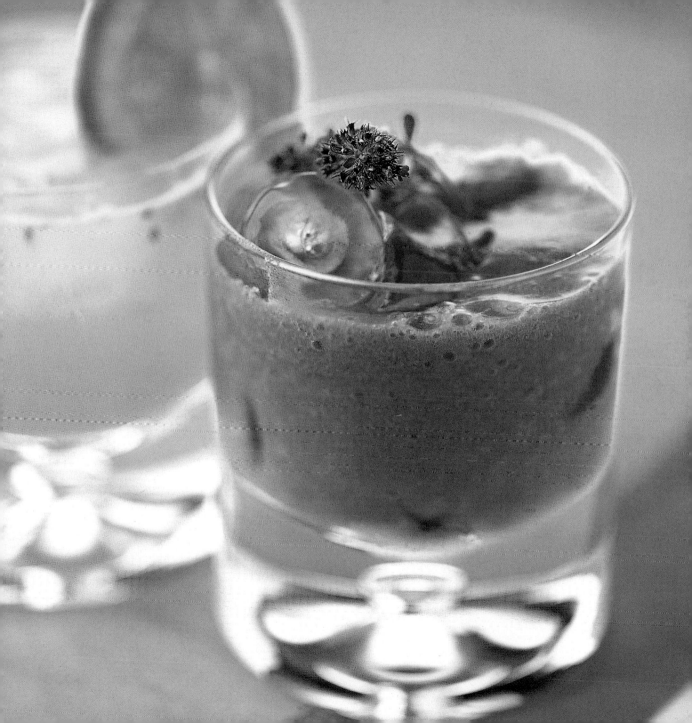

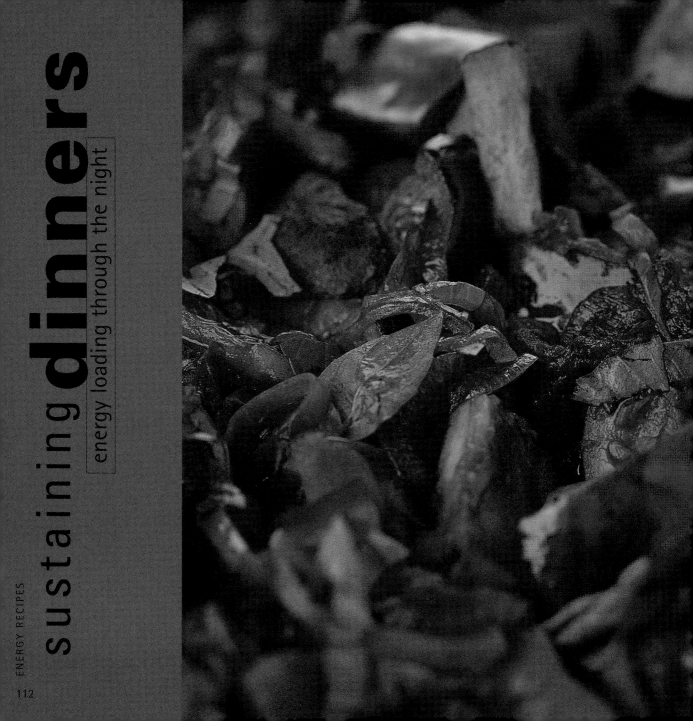

sustaining **dinners**

energy loading through the night

Ratatouille
with polenta cakes

Serves 4

Ratatouille

2 onions, sliced
5 tablespoons extra virgin olive oil
2 small eggplants, chopped
2 small zucchini, sliced
1 red pepper, sliced
1 green pepper, sliced
2 cloves of garlic, crushed
8 medium, ripe tomatoes, peeled
  and chopped
1 small bunch fresh basil, chopped
  (but keep some leaves whole for garnish)
Water
Sea salt and pepper
Tomato paste

1. Sauté the onions in the olive oil and add the other vegetables one at a time in the order given above.
2. Stir in the basil (keeping a few leaves to garnish the dish) and cook for two more minutes, adding extra water if required.
3. Season with salt and pepper, turn down the heat, cover and simmer gently for approximately 20 minutes.
4. Remove the lid and simmer for a further 5 minutes, thickening with a little tomato paste. Garnish with fresh basil.

Polenta cakes

Makes 12 cakes

2 cups pre-cooked polenta
2 teaspoons herbes de Provence
$1/2$ teaspoon sea salt
Pinch of black pepper
$1 1/4$ cups boiling water
Grapeseed oil

1. Put the polenta in a bowl, add the herbs, salt, pepper and mix well.
2. Gradually pour in the boiling water and stir to form a thick batter. Leave for 5 minutes, then knead to an even consistency.
3. Break off handfuls of the batter and mold them into small round cakes, 2 in in diameter by $1/2$ in thick.
4. Shallow-fry the cakes in a little oil until golden brown, turning frequently.
5. Serve with the ratatouille and thick slices of fresh bread.

Energy boost:	✪ ✪ ✪ ✪ ✪
Nutrients:	Vitamins A, C, E & B-group; calcium, iron, magnesium, selenium, zinc; essential fatty acids
Body benefits:	Immune & digestive systems

Carrot and almond jacket potatoes
with herb salad

Serves 4

Carrot and almond jacket potatoes
4 large baking potatoes
2 tablespoons extra virgin olive oil
4 large carrots, julienned
1 cup almonds, chopped
1 teaspoon orange zest
1 teaspoon maple syrup
Sea salt and pepper to taste

1. Wash and dry the potatoes and rub in a little olive oil.
2. Pierce them a few times with a fork and bake in a pre-heated oven at 400°F for approximately 75 minutes or until flesh is soft.
3. Put the rest of the olive oil in a skillet, add the julienned carrots and sauté gently for a few minutes.
4. Add the almonds and cook for another 2 minutes.
5. Add the orange zest, maple syrup, salt and pepper to taste.
6. Turn the heat down as low as possible and simmer until the carrots soften.
7. When the potatoes are cooked, remove them from the oven and cut a deep cross in the top of each one.
8. Gently open out the potatoes by pressing on the four slits of the cross, sprinkle a little sea salt onto the flesh and add some of the carrot and almond mixture.
9. Serve with herb salad and tarragon dressing.

Herb salad
1 small head of red-leaf lettuce, shredded
6–8 sorrel leaves, chopped
Handful of beet leaves, chopped
Bunch of cilantro, chopped
6–8 dandelion leaves (or Belgian endive), chopped

Mix all the ingredients together in a salad bowl and serve with tarragon dressing.

Tarragon dressing
3 tablespoons lemon juice
1 stalk fresh tarragon
$1/4$ teaspoon salt
1 clove garlic
$1/3$ cup safflower oil
Extra virgin olive oil to taste
Pinch of pepper

Put all the ingredients (except for the olive oil) in a blender and blend for 30 seconds. Add the olive oil to taste.

Energy boost:	✪ ✪ ✪	
Nutrients:	Vitamins C & E; calcium, iron; essential fatty acids	
Body benefits:	Heart; circulatory system	

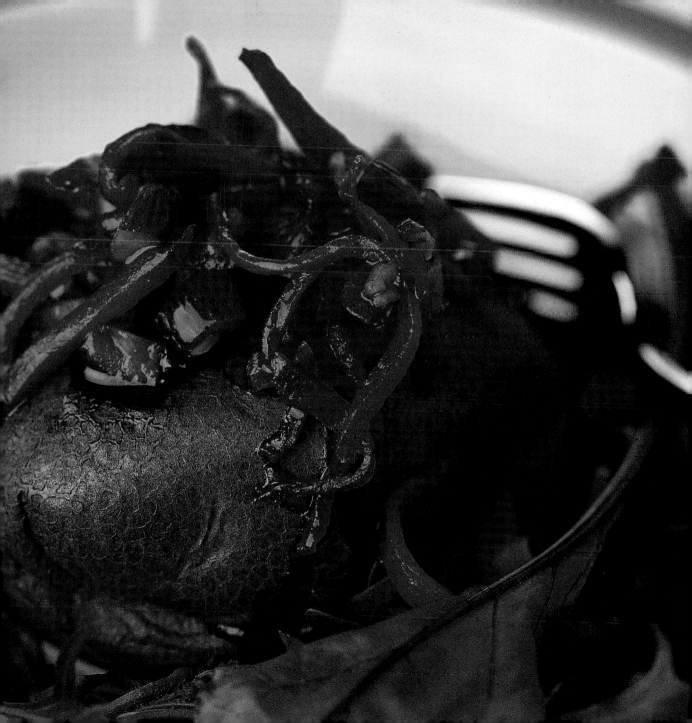

Aloo gobi

Serves 4

2 tablespoons extra virgin olive oil
Pinch of asafetida
1 teaspoon turmeric
$^1/_2$ teaspoon cayenne pepper
1 teaspoon ground cumin
3 tomatoes, peeled and chopped
1 tablespoon maple syrup
$^1/_2$ teaspoon sea salt
1 cup water
1 lb potatoes, quartered
1 medium cauliflower, separated into flowerets
1 teaspoon garam masala

1. Heat the oil in a large, heavy casserole, wok or karai, add the asafetida, turmeric, cayenne and cumin and sauté for a few seconds.
2. Add the tomatoes, maple syrup and salt and cook for a further minute.
3. Pour in the water, bring to a boil and add the potatoes, then cover and simmer for 10 minutes.
4. Add the cauliflower, bring back to a boil and simmer for a further 5 minutes (or until the vegetables are tender).
5. Sprinkle with garam masala and serve with basmati rice cooked in coconut milk with cumin and lime juice.

Energy boost:	✪ ✪ ✪ ✪
Nutrients:	Vitamins C, E, niacin, B$_6$ & folate; iron
Body benefits:	Immune & circulatory systems; skin

Vegetable crumble

Serves 4

2 cups plain flour
2 tablespoons flaked almonds
$^1/_2$ cup vegetable margarine
1 onion, sliced
2 medium carrots, sliced
2 stalks celery, sliced
$^1/_4$ cabbage, shredded
2 cups filberts, chopped
1 tablespoon yeast extract dissolved in $^3/_4$ cup
  boiling water
4 medium tomatoes, peeled and chopped
Sea salt and pepper to taste; flaked almonds to garnish

1. For the crumble, blend the flour with the almonds and half the margarine, keeping a tablespoon of flour aside.
2. Melt the rest of the margarine in a large pan and gently sauté the onions, carrots, celery and cabbage until soft. Add the filberts and heat through. Stir in the remaining flour.
3. Pour in the yeast extract mixture. Stir until it thickens.
4. Add the tomatoes, season with salt and pepper, and pour into a greased casserole dish.
5. Sprinkle the crumble mixture on top, garnish with flaked almonds and cook in the oven for approximately one hour at 350°F, until golden brown.
6. Serve with steamed haricots verts and corn.

Energy boost:	✪ ✪ ✪ ✪ ✪
Nutrients:	B-group vitamins; calcium, iron
Body benefits:	Immune & circulatory systems; bones; soft tissues; anti-stress

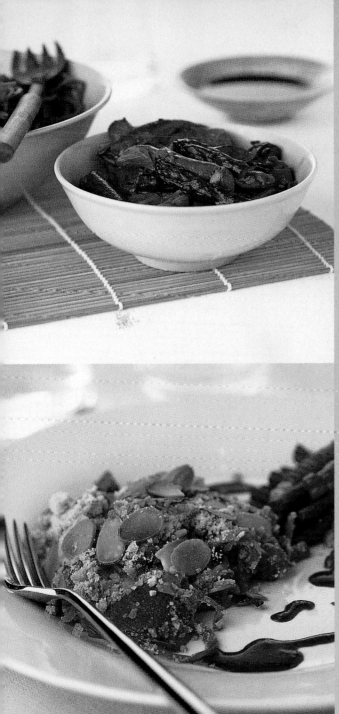

Asparagus, bean curd and mushrooms

Serves 4

2 tablespoons extra virgin olive oil

1 cup bean curd (tofu), diced

1 small leek, sliced

12 oyster mushrooms, cleaned and whole

1 clove garlic, crushed

1 teaspoon fresh ginger, finely chopped

1 bunch green asparagus, cut into small pieces
(discard the bottom 2 in of the stalks)

$^1/_3$ cup vegetable stock or water

2 tablespoons soy sauce; 2 tablespoons dry sherry

1 teaspoon cornstarch, dissolved in a little warm water

1. Heat the oil in a wok or large skillet and stir-fry the bean curd for a couple of minutes.

2. Add the leek and stir for another minute, then the mushrooms, garlic and ginger, stir-frying until the mushrooms release their moisture.

3. Add the asparagus, stock, soy sauce and sherry, then cover and simmer very gently until the asparagus is tender.

4. Add the cornstarch and stir until the sauce thickens.

5. Serve with noodles.

Energy boost:	✪ ✪ ✪ ✪
Nutrients:	Niacin, folate & biotin; calcium, iron, magnesium, zinc
Body benefits:	Immune, circulatory & nervous systems; skin & hair; bones & soft tissues

Spinach parcels
with onion sauce

Serves 4

Spinach parcels

1 lb fresh spinach

2 tablespoons olive oil

1 cup bean curd (tofu), diced

4 small green onions, finely chopped

1 clove garlic, finely chopped

1 tablespoon soy sauce

$^1/_2$ teaspoon crushed coriander seeds

$^1/_2$ teaspoon crushed cumin seeds

Sea salt and pepper to taste

1 packet strudel dough sheets

1. Wash the spinach and place, wet, in a large saucepan over a moderate heat, without adding further water. The spinach will steam in the water left on the leaves after rinsing.

2. When the leaves soften, remove them from the pan with a slotted spoon and chop them.

3. Heat the oil in a skillet and sauté the bean curd for 2–3 minutes. Add the green onions and the garlic, then the soy sauce, and cook for a minute before adding the spinach, coriander seeds and cumin.

4. Heat through and add sea salt and pepper to taste, then remove from heat.

5. Open out a sheet of strudel dough, brush with olive oil and place two generous spoonfuls of the spinach filling in the middle of the sheet.

6. Fold sheet into a parcel and repeat steps 6–7 until you have used up all the filling, then brush each parcel with oil.

7. Bake at 425°F, until golden.

8. Serve with onion sauce, new potatoes, peas and carrots.

Onion sauce

2 tablespoons olive oil

3 medium onions, finely chopped

2 tablespoons soy sauce

2 tablespoons wheat flour

$1^1/_3$ cups vegetable stock

$^1/_3$ cup soy milk

Sea salt and pepper to taste

1. Heat the oil gently in a casserole.

2. Add the onions and soften without allowing to brown.

3. Put in the soy sauce and wheat flour; stir well.

4. Gradually pour in the stock, stirring continuously, then simmer for a few minutes.

5. Add the soy milk, still stirring, and heat through.

6. Season with salt and pepper, and serve.

Energy boost:	✪ ✪ ✪ ✪
Nutrients:	Vitamins C, niacin, folate & pantothenate; calcium
Body benefits:	Nervous system; anti-stress

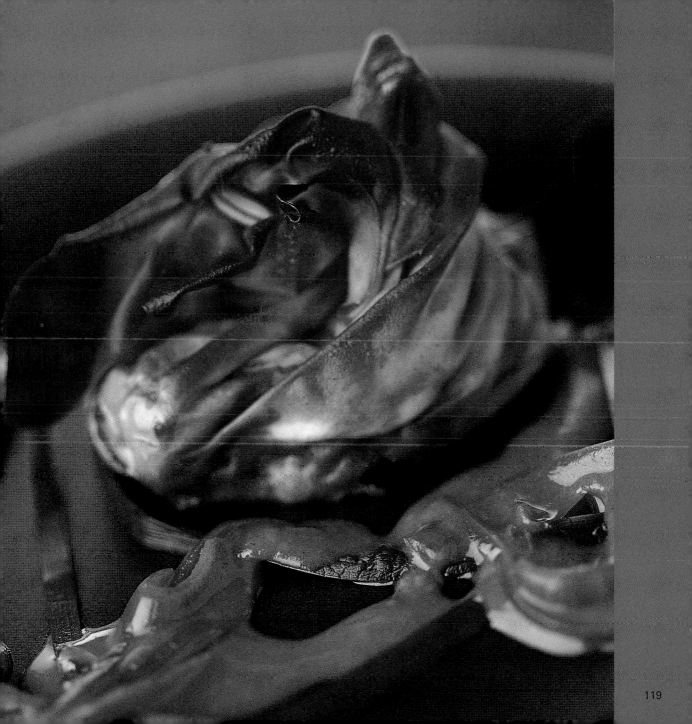

Sweet potato and hiziki

Serves 4

1 cup dried hiziki (seaweed)
4 tablespoons extra virgin olive oil
1 lb sweet potatoes, peeled and cut into thin sticks
$\frac{1}{3}$ cup vegetable stock
$\frac{1}{2}$ teaspoon sea salt
1 tablespoon maple syrup
1 tablespoon dry sherry
1 tablespoon soy sauce
1 tablespoon tahini

1. Rinse the seaweed in cold water.
2. Put in a bowl and cover with hot water.
3. Leave to soak for 15–20 minutes, adding more hot water from time to time to keep the seaweed completely immersed.
4. Discard the soaking water and rinse again.
5. Heat the oil gently in a wok or big pot.
6. Add the sweet potato and stir-fry for a few minutes, then put in the seaweed and cook for a further two minutes.
7. Add the rest of the cooking ingredients and stir. Cover and simmer gently for 5 minutes.
8. Serve with a mixture of rice and wild rice.

Energy boost:	✪ ✪ ✪ ✪ ✪
Nutrients:	Vitamins A, E & B-group; iodine, iron
Body benefits:	Immune, endocrine & nervous systems; skin

Nettle and lasagne bake

Serves 4

Nettle and lasagne bake

8 handfuls fresh young nettle tips – use gloves (if you have
  difficulty finding nettles, curly kale can be used instead)
1 onion, finely chopped
1 carrot, finely chopped
2¼ cups mushrooms, chopped
2 stalks celery, finely sliced
2 tablespoons extra virgin olive oil
4 tomatoes, peeled and chopped
1 teaspoon lemon juice
1 sprig fresh thyme, finely chopped (or ½ teaspoon dried)
1 bay leaf
Tomato paste
Sea salt and pepper to taste
1 packet lasagne sheets ("no pre-cooking required" variety)

1. Pick and wash the nettles using gloves, then steam in a
little water until soft. Remove from the pan and chop finely.
2. Sauté the onion, carrot, mushrooms and celery in the oil,
then add the steamed nettles, tomatoes, lemon juice, herbs
and a little tomato paste.
3. Simmer for about 5 minutes, or until mixture thickens.
4. Set aside while you make the white sauce.

White sauce

1 tablespoon vegetable margarine
2 tablespoons wheat flour
⅔ cup soy milk
Pinch of freshly grated nutmeg; sea salt and pepper

1. Melt the margarine gently in a saucepan and add the flour,
stirring for a minute.
2. Add the soy milk a little at a time, stirring continuously.
3. Bring to a boil and simmer for a couple of minutes.
4. Add nutmeg, salt and pepper to taste.

Lasagne topping

1 cup bean curd (tofu)
3 tablespoons soy sauce
2 tablespoons olive oil
½ cup water
2 teaspoons mustard
Salt and pepper

Blend all the ingredients to a smooth paste.

To make up the dish

Grease an ovenproof dish and cover the bottom with a thin
layer of white sauce. Put a layer of pasta on top, then add
a layer of nettle filling. Continue layering in this sequence,
ending with a layer of pasta. Spread the topping over
the bake. Transfer to a hot oven (425°F) and bake for
approximately 25 minutes (or until the lasagne is soft). Serve
with chopped cucumber and mint, dressed in lemon juice.

Energy boost:	✪ ✪ ✪ ✪ ✪
Nutrients:	Vitamins A, C, niacin, folate & pantothenate; calcium, iron
Body benefits:	Immune & circulatory systems; bones; soft tissues; anti-stress

Serves 4

Stuffed mushrooms

12–16 large portobello mushrooms

3 tablespoons extra virgin olive oil

2 cloves garlic, finely chopped

1 shallot, finely chopped

1 sprig fresh (or $1/2$ teaspoon dried) rosemary, chopped

1 tablespoon soy sauce

4–5 tablespoons breadcrumbs

1 small bunch parsley, finely chopped

1. Remove the mushroom stalks and set them aside.

2. Scoop out the black gills inside the mushroom caps with a teaspoon and discard.

3. Place the caps upside down (edges upward) in an oiled oven-proof dish or baking pan.

4. Finely chop the mushroom stalks and sauté in olive oil for one minute.

5. Add the garlic and shallot, and heat through.

6. Put in the rosemary and soy sauce and simmer until the mushrooms release their moisture.

7. Add enough breadcrumbs to soak up the liquid, then remove from the heat and add the parsley.

8. Fill the mushroom caps with the mixture.

9. Bake for 5–10 minutes at 400°F until golden brown.

10. Serve with spiced peaches and steamed new potatoes.

Spiced peaches

4 big, ripe peaches, peeled, pitted and sliced

4 tablespoons maple syrup

2 tablespoons lemon juice

2 teaspoons ground, roasted cumin

$1/4$ teaspoon cayenne pepper

$1/2$ teaspoon sea salt

Black pepper to taste

1. Put the peaches in a serving bowl.

2. Mix the other ingredients together, except the black pepper, and pour over the peaches.

3. Sprinkle with black pepper and serve immediately.

Energy boost:	✪ ✪ ✪
Nutrients:	Vitamins C, folate & biotin; iron
Body benefits:	Immune & nervous systems; skin & hair; detoxifying

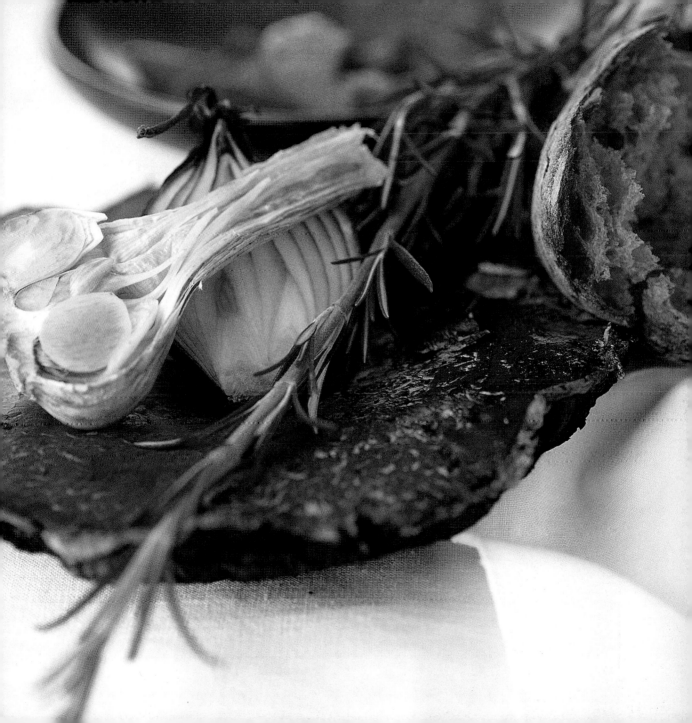

Dandelion coffee

You can buy dried dandelion roots from a healthfood store, or, between September and April, you can dig your own roots from the garden and dry them as follows:

2 or 3 dandelion roots

1. Wash the fresh roots and cut into short pieces.
2. Place on a baking pan in a warm oven (225–300°F) for several hours until completely dry.
3. Place the dried roots in a dry, heavy-weight skillet. Heat over a moderate heat.
4. Stir continuously until they turn a rich, dark brown.
5. Grind the roots in a coffee grinder. Store in a sealed container.
6. Brew and serve like regular coffee.

Body benefits:
Dandelion coffee is a renowned tonic for the liver and digestion. It also benefits the cardiovascular system and is detoxifying.

Anisette

1 star anise
2 sprigs of fresh lemon balm
Boiling water

1. Place the anise star and lemon balm sprigs in a cup.
2. Pour boiling water over to fill cup.
3. Leave to infuse for 5 minutes.
4. Remove one of the lemon balm sprigs and serve immediately.

Body benefits:
Star anise, a general stimulant, benefits the lungs as well as digestion, while the lemon balm relaxes the body and raises the spirits.

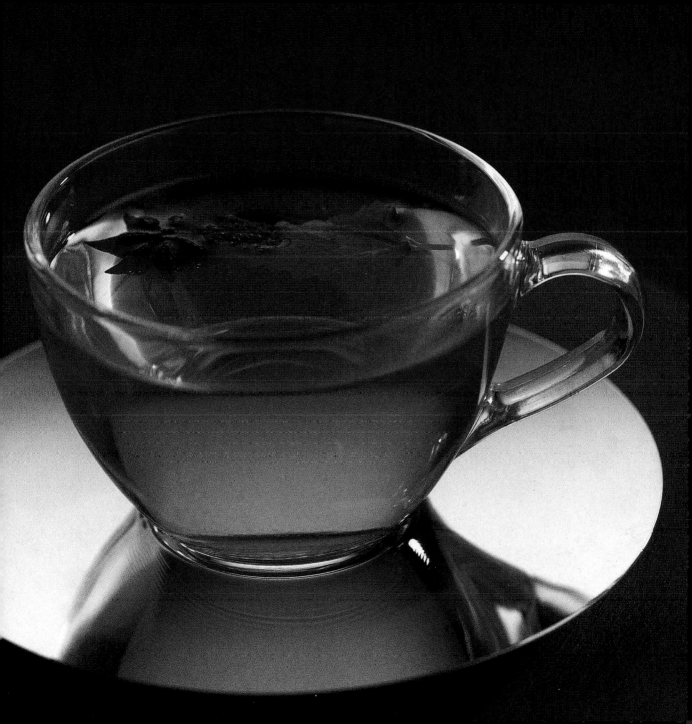

Sweet fennel

Sweet fennel is a relaxing and sweet-smelling aromatic herb, and a soothing digestive remedy suitable for all ages. It is traditionally said to increase the flow of milk in breast feeding mothers and, since its calming influence on the digestion passes to the baby with the breast milk, it also helps to ease infant colic.

Camomile flowers, with their distinctive scent of apples, are renowned for their gentle healing effects and for their ability to calm body, mind and spirit. Combined with sweet fennel and a little licorice, they make a delicious digestive drink that can be enjoyed at any time of day, and especially after meals.

$1/_2$ teaspoon fennel
$1/_2$ teaspoon camomile
$1/_2$ teaspoon licorice
1 cup boiling water

1. Place the herbs in a small, clean teapot.
2. Pour the cup of boiling water over them.
3. Leave to infuse for 5 minutes.
4. Strain and serve.

Body benefits:
This herbal blend has a soothing and calming effect on the digestion, gently relieving indigestion and colic. It also benefits the respiratory system.

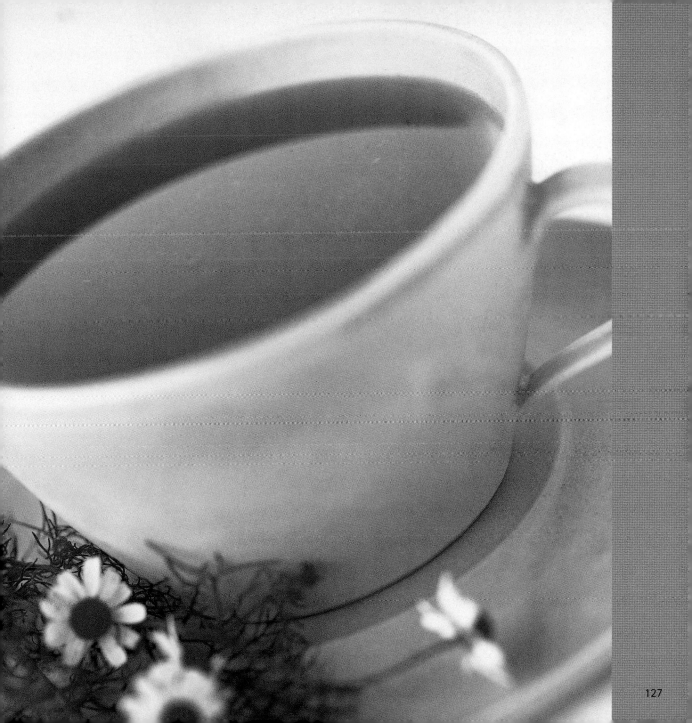

night caps

soothing drinks for healthy sleep

Sleepy time

$1/_2$ teaspoon camomile flowers
$1/_2$ teaspoon cowslip flowers
$1/_2$ teaspoon lime flowers
1 cup boiling water

1. Put the herbs in a small teapot.
2. Add the boiling water.
3. Cover and leave to infuse for
5–10 minutes.
4. Strain and serve.

Body benefits:

> This relaxing herbal blend benefits the digestive and nervous systems. Its anti-stress and mildly sedative properties naturally encourage restful sleep.

Hot cinnamon

$1^3/_4$ in long piece of cinnamon
 (or 1 teaspoon ground)
1 cup rice milk
1 teaspoon honey

1. Place the cinnamon and rice milk in a small saucepan. Bring to a boil.
2. Simmer for 2 minutes.
3. Pour into a mug and add the honey.
4. Drink immediately.

Body benefits:

> A warming and soothing bedtime drink which also aids digestion.

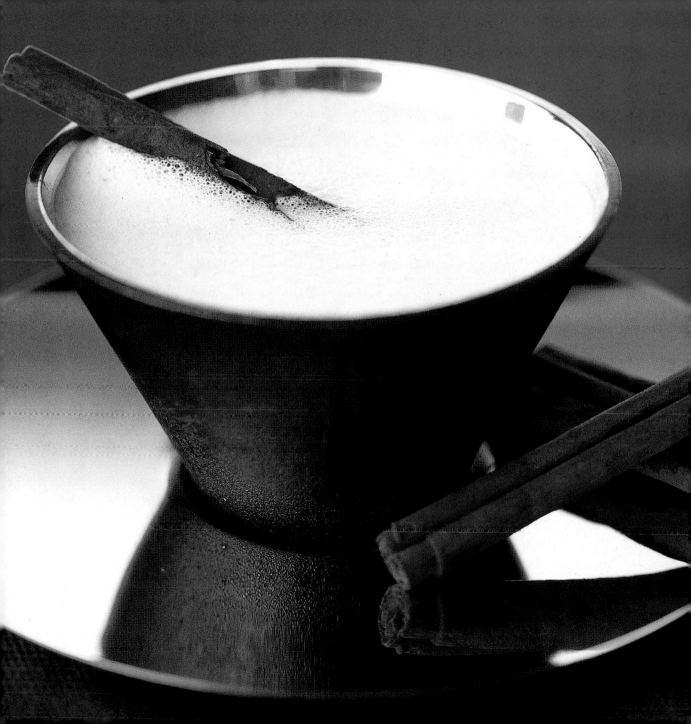

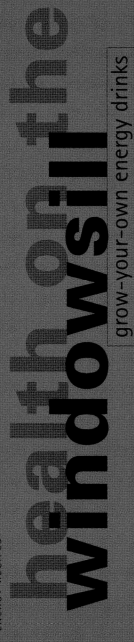

health on the windowsill

grow-your-own energy drinks

Thyme

A native of sundrenched mountain slopes, thyme thrives on warmth and well-drained soil. It makes an excellent aromatic tea with a warm, clove-like flavor.

A few young thyme shoots
1 cup boiling water

1. Place the thyme in a teapot.
2. Add the boiling water.
3. Leave to infuse for 5–10 minutes.
4. Strain and serve.

Body benefits:

Thyme benefits the digestive, respiratory and immune systems. Its antiseptic and antibiotic properties have been known and valued since ancient times.

Mint

Mint is particularly well suited to growing on a windowsill. Keep the soil moist and don't let it grow too tall – 6 in is about right. Mint tea soothes the digestion and stimulates the body and mind – the perfect after-meal pick-me-up.

A few leaf tips of mint
1 cup boiling water

1. Place the mint leaves in a teapot.
2. Add the boiling water.
3. Leave to infuse for 5–10 minutes.
4. Strain and serve.

Body benefits:

Mint, a general stimulant, benefits the nervous and immune systems. The cool, refreshing taste of fresh mint tea makes it a perfect after-dinner digestive.

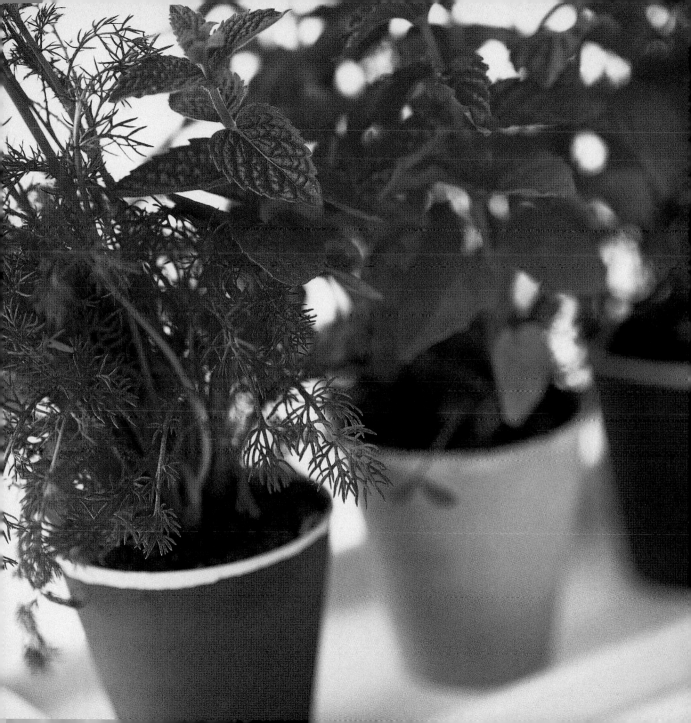

Vital force

9 oz fresh beet
$1/2$ in piece of fresh horseradish
$1/2$ grapefruit

1. Juice all three ingredients
and mix well.
2. Pour into a small tumbler and
serve garnished with a little extra
grated horseradish.

Beet is widely used by herbalists and naturopaths to
help relieve chronic illness and increase vitality.

Energy boost:	✪ ✪ ✪ ✪
Nutrients:	Vitamins C & folate; copper, iron, magnesium, zinc
Body benefits:	Immune system; blood; tissue-healing; blood fats; detoxifying

Deep heat

1 thick slice of lemon
1 piece of fresh ginger, $2/3$ in
  long, peeled and bruised
1 cup boiling water

1. Place the lemon and ginger in a
cup or rice bowl.
2. Add the boiling water and leave to
infuse for 2 minutes.
3. Remove the lemon and ginger with
a spoon. Drink immediately.

Known as the "garlic of the East", ginger is a natural
antibiotic and circulatory stimulant.

Energy boost:	✪ ✪ ✪
Nutrients:	Vitamins B_3 & C; calcium, magnesium, potassium
Body benefits:	Immune, digestive & cardiovascular systems

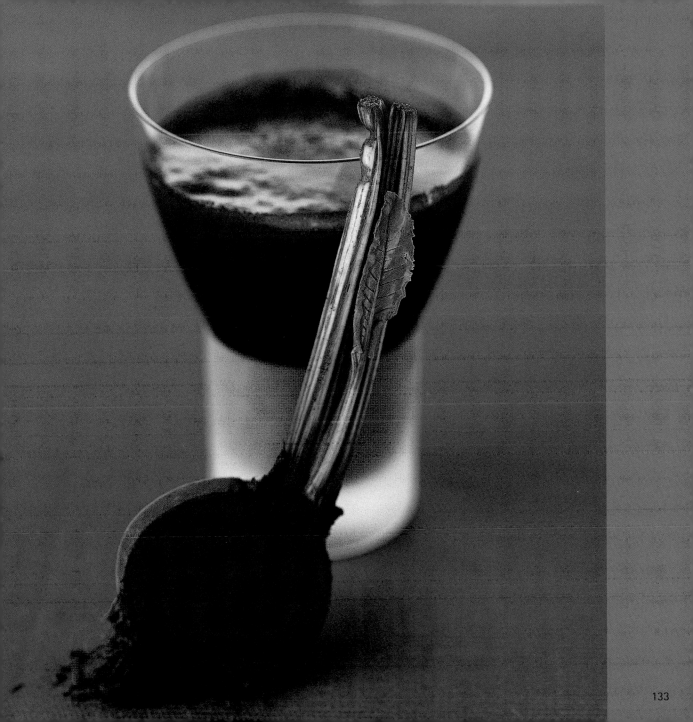

A plus

17$^1/_2$ oz carrots
1 stalk celery
1 small bunch parsley

1. Juice all the ingredients together. Reserve some parsley for garnishing.
2. Serve in a tall glass with the reserved parsley sprinkled on top.

Energy boost:	✪ ✪ ✪ ✪
Nutrients:	Vitamins A, K, B$_1$ & folate; calcium, iron, manganese, phosphorus, selenium, zinc
Body benefits:	Immune, cardiovascular & nervous systems; tissue–healing; skin; bones & muscles; blood

High C

5 oz redcurrants
5 oz blackcurrants
2 tablespoons natural organic soy yogurt
1 pinch of fresh grated ginger

Blend all the ingredients together. Serve chilled.

Energy boost:	✪ ✪ ✪
Nutrients:	Vitamins B$_2$, C & biotin; calcium, magnesium, phosphorus, potassium
Body benefits:	Immune & nervous systems; skin & hair; mucous membranes; blood

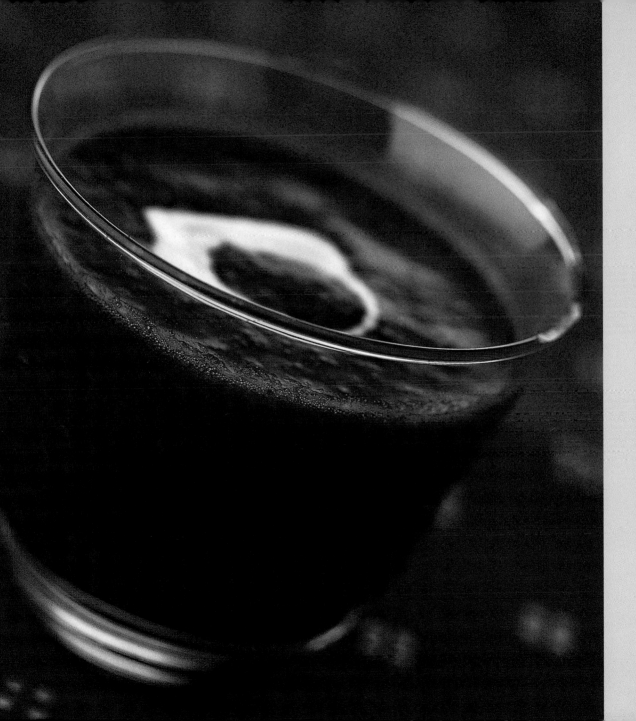

four seasons

timely juices throughout the year

Spring

1/2 cucumber	1 handful
1 scallion	dandelion leaves
2 carrots	1 pinch thyme
1 stalk celery	1 pinch salt

1. Juice the cucumber, scallion, carrots, celery and dandelion leaves.
2. Add the thyme and salt. Mix well.
3. Serve chilled.

Energy boost:	✪ ✪ ✪ ✪
Nutrients:	Vitamins A, K, B$_2$ & folate; calcium, iron, manganese, zinc
Body benefits:	Digestive, urinary & immune systems; detoxifying

Summer

Juice of 1/2 lemon	1/3 cup apple juice
A few lemon balm	1/3 cup fizzy water
sprigs	
A few mint sprigs	

1. Crush the herbs and add to the lemon juice. Pour into a tall glass.
2. Add the apple juice and fizzy water.
3. Serve chilled.

Energy boost:	✪ ✪ ✪
Nutrients:	Vitamins C, B$_3$ & folate; calcium, iron, magnesium
Body benefits:	Immune & nervous systems; skin; blood

Fall

1 bunch of muscat grapes
1 carrot
1 teaspoon filbert paste

1. Juice the grapes and the carrot.
2. Add the filbert paste and serve chilled.

Energy boost:	✪ ✪ ✪ ✪ ✪
Nutrients:	Vitamins A, E, K, B$_1$, B$_2$, B$_3$, biotin, B$_6$ & folate; calcium, copper, fluoride, iron, magnesium, manganese, phosphorus, potassium, zinc
Body benefits:	Whole-body nutritional workout

Winter

1 beet	1 pinch of cumin
1 carrot	1 small pinch salt
1 small leek	Ice cubes

1. Juice the beet, carrot and leek.
2. Add cumin and salt. Serve with ice.

Energy boost:	✪ ✪ ✪
Nutrients:	Vitamins A, K, B$_1$ & folate; calcium, copper, iron, magnesium, phosphorus, zinc
Body benefits:	Blood; immune & nervous systems; detoxifying

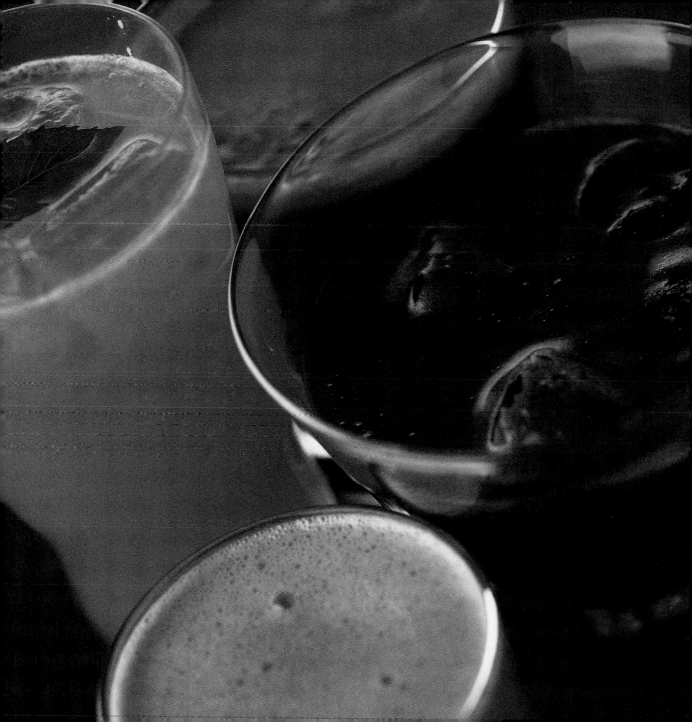

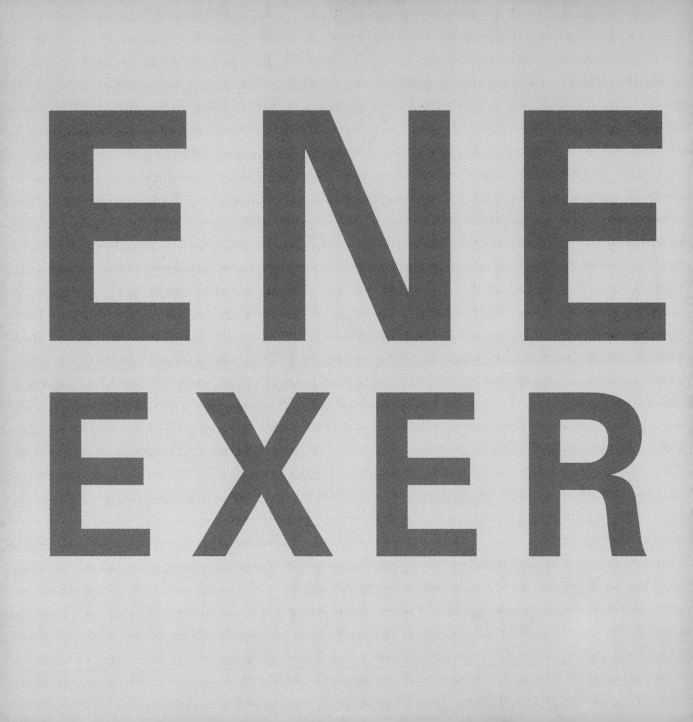

RGY
CISES

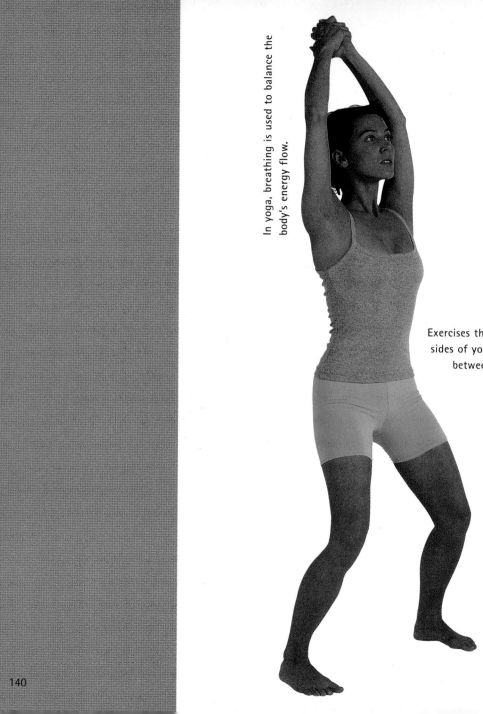

In yoga, breathing is used to balance the body's energy flow.

Exercises that balance the energy flow in both sides of your body stimulate the connections between the two sides of your brain.

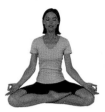

chapter five

Energy
balance

By stimulating the flow and restoring the natural balance of energy in our bodies, we can vastly improve the quality of our lives.

Energy flows through the body like a river and its tributaries, but often the stresses of Western living act like dams to cause flooding or drought, and disrupt the body's natural, harmonious state.

Imagine that you are able to summon up extra energy or switch off and relax at will. Imagine that your immune system reacts instantly to repel disease, and that you are nurtured with deep, nourishing sleep, and wake up feeling rejuvenated and eager to fulfill the potential of each day. When our body's energy flows freely and in balance, these benefits fall open to us.

Chinese wisdom

Balancing the flow of energy around the body has been the central aim of exercise disciplines throughout the Far East for centuries. In the Chinese traditions, energy flows along specific paths named meridians. There are said to be twelve meridians, each relating to a particular organ such as the stomach, the spleen, the kidneys and the liver. The body also has two reservoirs of energy known as vessels, which run up through the center of the torso and head (see p.145).

Energy is known as *qi* or *chi* (pronounced "chee") in China and is created by the tension between two opposing forces, "yin" and "yang". The male, yang energy is represented by the sun, and the female, yin energy is embodied in the earth.

There are three sources of *qi*. We receive congenital *qi*, which is stored in the kidneys, from both parents at conception. It is a barometer of our overall vitality, which can be depleted by stress, lack of sleep and stimulants – dark rings under the eyes are a sign of low congenital *qi*. Nutritive *qi* enters the body through the air we breathe and the food we eat. Protective *qi* surrounds our bodies. It prevents us suffering from excess cold or heat, and strengthens the immune system. To enjoy good health we need constantly to replenish our *qi* and encourage a strong, balanced flow around the body, by practicing energy exercises such as t'ai chi and qigong, and by breathing correctly, eating natural foods, drinking fresh water and benefitting from the right amount of sleep.

When we are affected by stress, shock, toxins or emotional problems, the meridians become blocked and this can cause imbalance in and impede the body's energy flow, in turn causing disease. This book includes some specific exercises for removing blockages (see pp.146–7).

Rivers of energy
the meridians

Each of our twelve meridians has two channels, one on each side of the body. The meridians form six pairs. One of each pair is a yin meridian, drawing up energy from the earth. This energy flows up the insides of the legs, up the body, and along the insides of the arms to the fingertips. The six yang meridians draw *qi* down from the sky, and the energy flows from the fingertips to the shoulders, head and body, and down the outsides of the legs.

Although we cannot see them, the meridians of the body can be measured electrically. Tests have led practitioners to believe that they are located just under the skin.

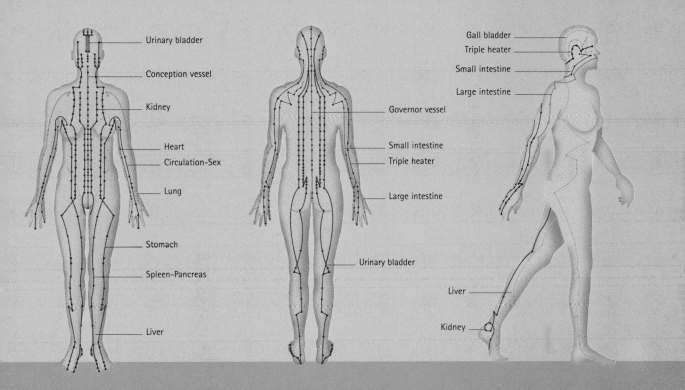

The meridians are all connected. The *qi* flows along them in a particular direction and around the body in a continuous cycle (see arrows in the key, right). The yin meridians are those of the lung, spleen-pancreas, heart, kidney, circulation-sex and liver; the corresponding yang meridians are those of the large intestine, stomach, small intestine, urinary bladder, triple heater and gall bladder.

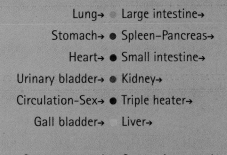

Lung→	●	Large intestine→
Stomach→	●	Spleen–Pancreas→
Heart→	●	Small intestine→
Urinary bladder→	●	Kidney→
Circulation-Sex→	●	Triple heater→
Gall bladder→		Liver→

Governor vessel ● Conception vessel

Unblocking the meridians

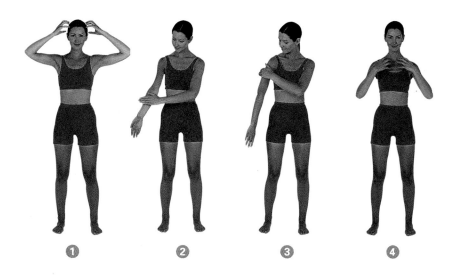

1 Tap all over your head with your fingertips, then stroke your hair. **2** Brush down the inside of each arm, from armpit to fingertips. **3** Brush up the outsides to the shoulders. **4** Tap your upper chest.

In this qigong exercise the hands sweep every meridian in the direction of the energy flow. In this way the movement of energy will break through any blockages, restoring balance and increasing vitality.

Launch into the day with this energy booster – it is especially good for banishing sluggishness in the morning.

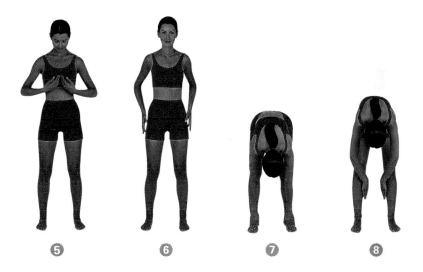

5 Run your fingertips down your breastbone. **6** Pat your hips and smooth down the outsides of your legs. **7** Pass your hands over your feet. **8** Continue up the insides of your legs. Repeat 10 times.

Qigong

The ancient Chinese tradition of qigong has a history stretching back more than 5,000 years. Today it is practiced by millions of Chinese to promote energy flow for health and spiritual wellbeing.

The word qigong is made up of two Chinese words: *qi*, meaning energy or vitality, and *gong*, meaning practice. Together they mean "repeated energy work" – the basic (if rather simplified) philosophy behind this Eastern tradition.

Stand, feet parallel, shoulders' width apart. Stretch your feet and splay out your toes. Your knees should be slightly bent and gently eased outward by your thighs. Gently draw up your abdominal muscles and allow your buttocks to sink toward the floor – from the waist down, your body should feel grounded. Lower your shoulders, drop your chin slightly to relax your neck, keeping your head erect as if it is being held from above. Let your arms hang down loosely, as if they were floating slightly outward. You should feel completely balanced and relaxed – if you feel any strain, try to ease it away as you breathe out.

Imagine that you are a tree. Visualize roots growing down from your feet, deep into the earth. You are tapping into the earth's goodness, which you draw up through your roots to nourish you. With each breath, you take in pure, positive energy to stimulate the flow of *qi* around your body and, as you exhale, you expel all the negative energy, toxins and anxieties into the earth, where they are absorbed and purified. You feel as if all your cares have melted away. Let your mind rest and feel at peace.

Qigong is said to be both subtle and internal: subtle because it is non-physical and intangible; internal because it focuses our energy inward.

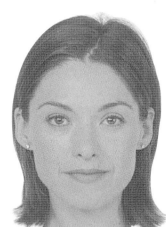

Achieving and maintaining balance

1 Adopt the Qigong Basic Posture (see p.149). Bring your elbows up and fingers in to the breastbone. **2** Reach out your arms; keep your shoulders relaxed and imagine wrapping your arms around a huge ball of energy. **3** Sweep your arms forward, squeezing the "ball"; bring your fingers back to your breastbone and drop your head forward. Repeat 15 times.

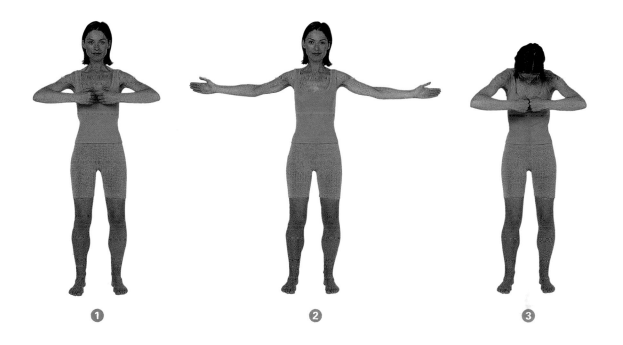

1

2

3

We often throw our bodies out of alignment by carrying a bag (or even our baby) with one arm, or standing with more weight on one leg, or always sleeping on one side. This exercise improves our bodies' symmetry, which opens up the central energy channel and balances energy flow around the whole body.

Ancient Chinese Daoists believed that a balanced flow of qi was the key to a long, healthy life.

Strengthening the energy flow

1 Stand, feet shoulders' width apart, knees slightly bent. Elbows out, bring your hands, palms inward, to your chest. **2** Stretch your arms out to the side. **3** Bring them up high above your head. **4** Cradle your skull in your hands. **5** Following the contors of your body, but without your palms actually touching your skin, sweep over your shoulders and down your chest to your lower ribs. **6** Sweep round to your back so that one hand is over each kidney. **7** Run your palms over your hips and down the outsides of your legs. Sweep round the front of your feet and up your inner calves and thighs, returning to the lower abdomen. Repeat 20 times.

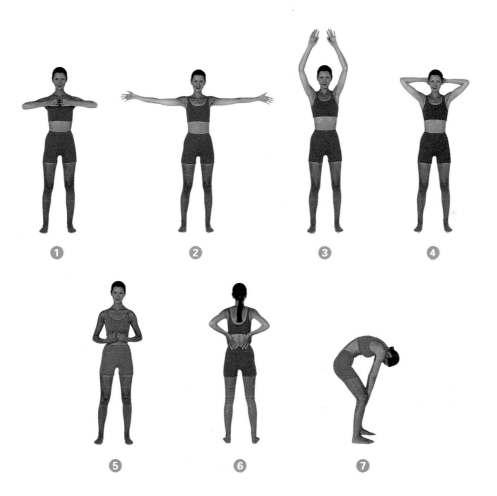

All meridian flow is stimulated by this qigong movement, but it particularly increases energy flow through the gall bladder (the outsides of the legs, hips and abdomen), the large intestine (the shoulders), and the liver, kidney and spleen-pancreas meridians, which run up the insides of the legs.

Sweep your body as the mood takes you: whether slow or quick, this exercise will keep your energy flowing strongly.

Visualizing energy

1 Standing with both feet planted firmly on the ground, cross your right leg over your left leg and your right arm over your left arm; now link your fingers together. **2** Keeping your fingers locked, twist your hands under and up, and at the same time press your tongue to the roof of your mouth. Breathe deeply, and visualize energy flowing around your body for one minute. **3** Keeping your tongue pressed into the roof of your mouth, uncross your arms and legs. Stand with your feet apart, bend your arms up and touch fingertips, then breathe deeply for one minute. Repeat the whole sequence, this time crossing your left leg over your right leg and your left arm over your right arm.

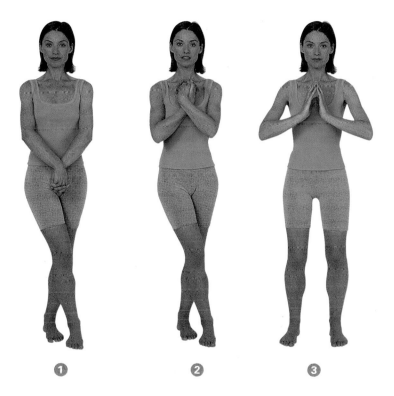

This kinesiology exercise, known as "Cook's Hook-up", is perfect to do first thing in the morning – it ensures that your energy flow is balanced from the very start of the day.

Go on! Kick-start your energy!

Our bodies have evolved so that they produce extra epinephrine when we are threatened. This makes our hearts pump more blood to our muscles to enable us to fight a predator or run away from danger. Today, we are more likely to face traffic jams than wild animals and, as aggression or escape are no longer appropriate responses, we tend to block the out-flow of excess energy, thus contributing to the build-up of stress. These exercises (pp.157–9) provide safe, alternative ways to release accumulated tension and re-establish your body's energy balance.

Fight or flight

the natural energy rush

"Comfort foods", such as candy, increase the levels of epinephrine in our bodies – don't be tempted!

The eyebrow squeeze

Move your thumbs along the bone behind your eyebrows to find a groove near to your nose. Press into this with the inside corner of your thumb. Squeeze your eyebrows between your thumbs and index fingers, moving from the nose outward.

The wood chopper

1 Stand, feet shoulders' width apart, knees bent. Clasp your hands together and lift your arms above your head, raising your chest and taking a deep breath. **2** Swing your arms down while exhaling and shouting "Ha!" as loudly as you can. **3** Keep the swing going until you have reached your arms as far through your legs as possible. **4** Swing your arms up again until they are high above your head. Repeat as many times as you feel are necessary to release any excess energy in your system.

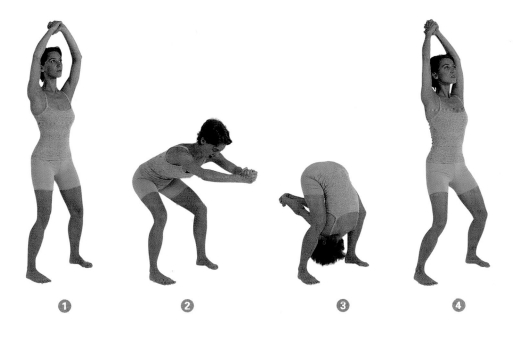

This polarity therapy exercise releases blocked energy from the solar plexus chakra (*manipura*), which if allowed to build up, can affect your judgment and cause indigestion.

Polarity therapy, developed by Dr. Randolph Stone (1890–1981), is a form of holistic healing, which treats the mind, body and spirit, and the energy system.

Paths to yoga

Yoga is a way of integrating the mind, body and spirit, leading you to a healthier and more fulfilled life. There are four main paths to yoga: Karma yoga (yoga of action), Bhakti yoga (yoga of devotion), Jnana yoga (yoga of knowledge) and Raja yoga (often called the "royal road"). Raja yoga is the mastery of mind and body in order to release the higher nature. Hatha yoga is widely practised in the West and is a sub-type of Raja yoga. Hatha yoga includes posture (*asana*), breathing (*pranayama*), meditation (*dhyana*) and cleansing practices (*shatkarmas*).

The various postures and breathing techniques that form the basis of the modern practice of Hatha yoga are contained in the classic 8th- and 9th-century text, *Hatha Yoga Pradipika*.

The *asanas* work on stretching and toning the muscles and skeletal framework of the body, as well as conditioning the organs and the nervous system. *Pranayama* practices calm the mind and revitalize the entire being. Relaxation and *dhyana* bring increased concentration and clarity. The cleansing practices of Hatha yoga, known as *shatkarmas* or *kriyas*, are very powerful and should be learnt only from a teacher.

Regularly practicing yoga helps to restore balance and harmony in the body and mind, removes toxins from the body and releases vast resources of untapped energy.

"Prior to everything, asana is spoken of as the first part of Hatha yoga." *Hatha Yoga Pradipika* (1:17)

Subtle anatomy

chakras and *nadis*

Western medicine tends to view the body as a collection of replaceable parts, many of which can be treated in isolation from one another. Other traditions view the body in a more holistic way, recognizing an essential inner energy, known as "life-force energy" or "vital force". In yoga teaching this energy is known as *prana*; when the balance of *prana* is disrupted, the result is illness. In yoga tradition the body has a system of chakras and *nadis* (channels) that generate and regulate *prana*. There are seven chakras on the midline of the body and many *nadis* through which *prana* flows.

"The removal of impurities allows the body to function more efficiently." *Yoga Sutras of Patanjali* (2:43)

Although chakras cannot be seen physically, they do have a relationship with the major physical organs in the body. They are positioned along the line of the spine. Many healers describe them as "spinning wheels of energy" and they are often represented by sound and color. The chakras are connected by three main *nadis*: *ida*, which passes by the left nostril; *pingala*, which passes by the right nostril; and *sushumna*, which runs up the middle of the spine. *Pranayama* and *asana* practice balances the flow of *prana*. Concentrating on certain chakras during *asana* practice can enhance the benefits of a posture.

- Crown chakra – *sahasrara*
- Third-eye chakra – *ajna*
- Throat chakra – *vishuddhi*
- Heart chakra – *anahata*
- Solar-plexus chakra – *manipura*
- Sacral chakra – *swadhisthana*
- Base chakra – *muladhara*

- Left side – *ida*
- Right side – *pingala*
- Center – *sushumna*

Moving to stillness

making contact with *purusa*

Most of us live in a stressful environment. Some stress is useful – it drives us to meet our goals. Most of us, however, add unnecessarily to the stress in our lives; we often rush to and from work on busy transport systems, we carry too many bags, and we sit and stand in ways that make the body stiff and misaligned. Whether we are at work or at home, we spend much time sitting in front of a computer or television screen. All of these things sap our energy. Although it is impossible to banish stress entirely, we can learn ways to manage it. A main aim of yoga is to find a place of spiritual stillness from which to respond to the world: achieving stillness in postures and mastering your breath are vital steps toward this.

People often start to practice yoga because they wish to change something in their lives: to feel more healthy, be more positive, think more clearly, be calmer or have more energy. This impetus for change ultimately comes from a place deep within us that yearns to be quiet and content and free from judgment and blame. In Sanskrit this spiritual place is known as *purusa*.

Yoga is not about striving for the impossible – that is, attempting to achieve incredibly complex postures before you are ready. It is about working within your limits and developing a personal practice that brings you into contact with your internal energy flow and self-awareness. By learning to direct energy through the use of breath, the body, mind and emotions will come into harmony. This in turn leads you to a place of quiet and stillness, where decisions can be made with clarity and insight. Once you make contact with this place of stillness, you will notice that stressful parts of your life become more manageable. Make a commitment to live your life responsibly, fully experiencing each moment from a quiet place of understanding: this is yoga.

"The mind can reach the state of yoga through tireless endeavor and non-attachment." *Yoga Sutras of Patanjali* (1:12)

Relaxation posture

Shavasana is one of the most important *asanas* in yoga. You can use it to center yourself at the start of a yoga practice, and at the end as a final relaxation. You can also use it as a resting posture between more dynamic *asanas*. It is called the corpse pose because it requires you to lie perfectly still, and to slow your breath. This helps the mind to become quiet. Once you have mastered this posture, you can use it to relax at any time.

Lie down on your back, preferably on a blanket or a mat. You may need a folded blanket underneath your head for comfort. Visualize an imaginary line running from the top of your head to between your feet. Your body should be lying equally on either side of this line. Your hands should be about 6 in away from your body with your palms facing upward. Your feet should be 12–16 in apart. Lift your pelvis and lightly reposition it to let the spine lengthen. Allow each vertebra to relax and sink into the floor. Check that your head is straight and not to one side.

Now relax completely, knowing that your body and being are supported. Concentrate on the tip of your nose and focus on the breath as it enters and leaves the nostrils. Follow the breath up your nose then down into your throat and lungs. Imagine that you are floating above yourself, observing your body lying on the floor. Breathe "into" any points of tension, allowing them to dissolve. Finally, bring your awareness back to the tip of your nose. Think to yourself: "I know I am breathing in, I know I am breathing out."

If you have lower-back problems, you can make this pose more comfortable by putting a bolster or cushion under your knees.

Simply sitting

Dandasana, the staff pose

Dandasana is the root of several other sitting postures. It might look deceptively easy, but to perfect it requires vigorous attention to detail. The legs and the torso form a right angle, the chest is expanded and the shoulders are relaxed. At the same time, your breath should flow easily and help you feel revitalized. Your face and jaw should be completely relaxed.

Sit with your legs stretched out in front of you. Place your hands on the floor by your hips, either with your palms flat or on your fingertips. Supporting yourself on your hands, lift your hips off the floor and move the base of your spine back a little before lowering yourself again. You should now feel solidly rooted to the ground. Tighten your knees and stretch your heels away from you, with your ankles gently flexed and your toes pointing upward.

Press down on your fingertips and breathe in. Extend your spine upward, lengthen your lower back and imagine the top of your head is held on a fine thread. Open your chest area and lift your shoulders up and back. Breathe out. Let your eye muscles relax so that your focus is soft (or close your eyes). Now relax your jaw, cheeks, forehead and scalp. Release any remaining tension on each out-breath.

Raise your arms and make your hands into fists with your thumbs enclosed in your fingers. Breathe in. As you breathe out, flick your fingers outward, stretching them as far as you can. Then bring your fingers to the floor or fold your hands in your lap and return your awareness to your breathing.

Learning to sit without discomfort is fundamental to good yoga practice.

Standing tall

Tadasana, the mountain pose

We often overlook the energy-giving potential of everyday postures. Even an apparently simple standing position such as *tadasana* can be invigorating. The mountain pose helps to release tension that builds up imperceptibly in our bodies throughout the day. It may be considered one of the most fundamental *asanas* – the point of departure not just for the other standing postures, but for all yoga postures.

The idea of the mountain suggests stillness, strength and steadfastness – all crucial elements of yoga practice.

Stand with your feet close together, the inside edges parallel and nearly touching. If this is uncomfortable, move them apart slightly. Take your awareness down to the soles of your feet and feel the connection with the ground. Spread your toes. Shift your weight back a little and ensure that your heels are firmly on the floor. Imagine that you have strong roots that reach down from your feet into the earth, enabling you to draw energy up into your body, as with the Qigong Basic Posture on page 149. Visualize the energy flow as you tighten and relax each group of muscles and ligaments in turn: first the ankles, then the calves, knees (you may need to bend them slightly), thighs and hips.

Take a deep breath and, as you exhale, check that your lower limbs are relaxed. Tip your hips forward slightly, while gently pulling the abdominal muscles upward. Move your awareness to your diaphragm, chest and shoulders, and tense and relax each in turn. Take another deep breath in and raise your shoulders toward your ears. On your out-breath allow your shoulders to drop and relax. Imagine a fine thread gently pulling you by the top of the head toward the sky. Inhale, then say "ha" as you let the air out. Finally, bring your hands together in front of your chest in the prayer position, and breathe in and out, not controlling the breath but simply letting it flow.

Yoga breathing
Pranayama

The key to releasing energy through yoga practice lies in the use of the breath. Because breathing is an automatic process, most of the time we are not aware of it and do not breathe to full capacity. *Pranayama* practice focuses awareness on the breath and the ability of pranic energy to revitalize the being. Most movements in *asana* practice are linked to in-breaths and out-breaths. Try to breathe through your nose, synchronizing each breath with the movement of your body.

Prana **means "vital force" or "life-force energy";** ayama **is defined as "expansion".**

Sit in a comfortable cross-legged position, press your palms on the floor and extend your spine upward, opening your chest. Place your palms on your knees.

Then place one hand on your abdomen at the level of the navel and breathe in slowly and deeply, allowing the abdomen to balloon outward. Breathe out slowly, using the abdominal muscles to contract the abdomen and expel all the remaining air. Repeat twice.

Now move both hands to the bottom of the ribcage so that the middle fingertips lie touching one another along the line of the lowest rib. Breathe in, expanding the ribcage as far as possible to the front, back and sides. Notice how far the fingers separate. (Check this again after a few months – you may find your lung capacity has increased.) Repeat twice.

Cross your arms and place your fingertips just below your collarbones. Breathe into the area at the top of the lungs, letting the breath come up as high as possible without straining. Let any tension drop away from your jaw or neck. Repeat twice. Now try to put the 3 actions together: breathe slowly and smoothly into the abdomen, ribcage and the top of the chest in one continuous inhalation. Then release the breath from the body. Repeat up to 5 times.

"Having gained control of the body through asana practice, pranayamas should be practiced." *Hatha Yoga Pradipika (2:1)*

Warming the body

Pawanmuktasanas

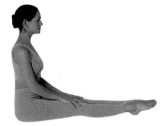

Toe and ankle flex

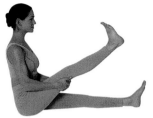

Knee bend

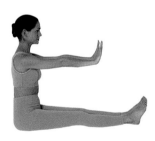

Wrist bend

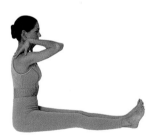

Shoulder rotation

These warm-ups prepare the body for more dynamic postures by releasing energy blockages in joints and muscles. They can also help to alleviate rheumatism and arthritis, and are excellent for people who are advised not to practice more strenuous postures.

You can do these postures at home or at work, sitting on a chair or sitting on the floor – whichever is easier.

Toe and ankle flex Breathe in and curl your toes back toward your body. Breathe out and curl them away. Repeat 5 times. Now do the same with your entire foot.

Knee bend Lift your right leg with both hands under the back of the knee. Breathe in and straighten your leg. Breathe out and bend your leg. Do not let your heel touch the floor. Repeat 5 times and then change legs.

Wrist bend Stretch your arms out in front. Breathe in and bend your hands back at the wrists. Breathe out and extend them forward and down. Repeat 5 times.

Shoulder rotation With your fingertips on the tops of your shoulders, rotate your elbows in a small circle. Make the circle bigger and include the shoulders in the movement. Breathe in as your elbows rise and out as they drop. Repeat 5 times then reverse direction.

Be bendy! The winning formula for maximizing the body's potential is said to be the flexibility of a child ...

... combined with an adult's mental and physical strength.

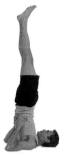

chapter six

Flexibility and motion

When we are conscious of our body's energies, we realize that during movement we are using energy to create more energy.

In the West the idea of exercise conjures up images of activities

such as high-impact aerobics or jogging. Such strenuous workouts

can impose stress on the body's joints and cardiovascular system.

As a result, gentler types of exercise such as yoga, qigong and

t'ai chi, which involve the use of static or slow-moving postures,

and require mental as well as physical discipline, are gaining in

popularity. Traditions such as these stimulate energy flow and make

our movements more fluid as well as improving our overall fitness

– without all the huffing, puffing and exhaustion.

The waist swing

Much of the enjoyment in this t'ai chi exercise stems from
the graceful, rhythmical movement that increases energy flow.
It relaxes the upper body and calms the mind while toning the
abdominal muscles and massaging the internal organs.

Swing away stress! This exercise will loosen your shoulders and trim your waist.

❶ Stand, feet hips' width apart and flat on the ground, knees loose. Keeping the upper body relaxed and the arms floppy, thrust your right hipbone forward and your left hipbone back. **❷** Return the swing by pushing your left hipbone forward and your right hipbone back. The twisting motion encourages the shoulders to follow and the arms to swing of their own accord. Concentrate on the hip motion and keep the upper body fluid. Continue until you feel warm and relaxed.

Pushing and pulling

1 Stand, feet shoulders' width apart. Inhale, raising your left elbow upward and parallel to the ground, the palm of your hand facing your chest. Raise your right forearm vertically, palm facing forward. Put your palms together. **2** Step forward with your left foot, pressing your right hand against the left, pushing the left hand forward beyond your foot as you exhale. **3** Use your left hand to pull the right one back. Inhale and bring your weight back onto your right foot. **4** Stand, feet parallel, shoulders' width apart. Elbows bent, open your arms with your palms facing forward and exhale. Repeat the whole sequence slowly, 5 times. Swap over to the other side.

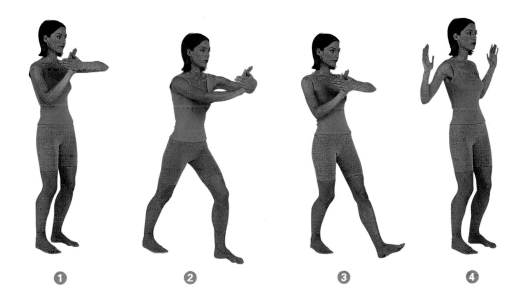

This t'ai chi exercise promotes the sensitive, flowing and reciprocal motion of energies between the hands. It encourages awareness of the interplay between the opposing yet complementary forces of yin and yang (for example, through pushing and pulling, controlling and yielding, giving and receiving) and it helps to restore balance between the two forces.

Practitioners of t'ai chi often benefit from a high level of flexibility well into old age – the gentle movements mean that the exercises can be done by anyone, at any time of life.

Movement to strengthen the legs

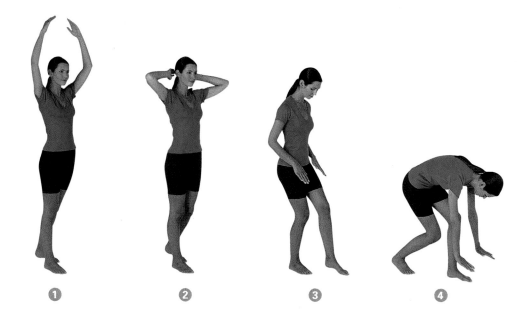

This qigong walking exercise grounds the body's energy, promoting a good flow. It tones the muscles in the legs, shoulders and arms, and encourages increased flexibility and coordination.

According to the principles of qigong, each time we place a foot on the ground when we walk, we are reconnecting with the vital energies of the earth.

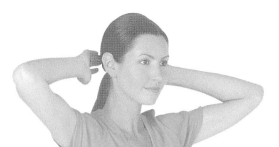

1 Step forward, put your weight on your right foot, your arms curved above your head. **2** As you begin to move your left foot forward, put your hands behind your head. **3** Sweep your hands over your shoulders and down to hip level as you move your left foot in front of your right and transfer weight onto it. **4** Lean forward at your waist, bend your knees and move your hands as far as you can toward the floor. Repeat 10 times, then swap legs.

Egyptian figures of eight

1 Stand, feet a little more than hips' width apart, firmly on the ground. **2** Keeping your knees slightly bent, move your right hip forward. **3** Push your right hip out to the side and then back, in a smooth circular motion. **4** Without hesitating, move your left hip forward. **5** Push your left hip out to the side and then back. Repeat, leading with alternate hips as if you are outlining a figure of eight. Maintain a rhythm, focusing on fluidly moving your hips while keeping your spine upright. Move your arms in the air to improve balance and add elegance.

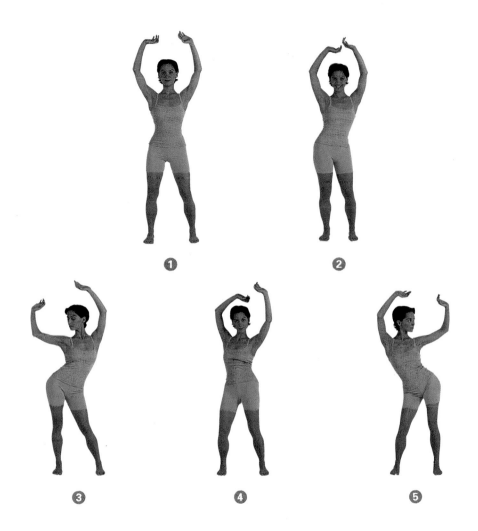

In Egyptian (or belly) dancing, the hips and abdomen move vigorously, leading the rest of the body, while the feet stay still – in this way the dancer maintains a connection with earth energies. Belly dancing tones the waist and hip areas and increases their flexibility. It also helps to heal pelvic, urinary, gynecological and digestive disorders.

"As long as there is life, there will be dance." (Margaret N. H. Doubler)

Egyptian hip drops

1 Stand with your feet hips' width apart, your right foot slightly forward. Keep your back and shoulders relaxed. Bend your left knee a little and raise your right heel, keeping the ball of your foot and your toes firmly on the ground. **2** Using your toes to push up, lift your right hip. **3** Bring the right hip forward and then lower it. Allow your arms, held above your head, to flow with the hip movement. **4** Sweep your right hip in a circle, from the front to the side and then back. Repeat Steps 2–4. Continue this sweeping motion for as long as you wish in a rhythmical and smooth movement. Repeat with your left hip for the same amount of time.

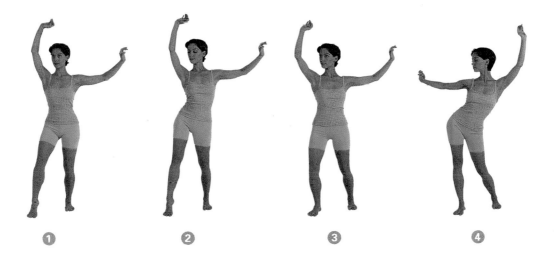

In this Egyptian dance exercise, energy flow is improved in the kidney, liver, urinary bladder, gall bladder, stomach and spleen-pancreas meridians, all of which pass through the pelvic area. Hip drops tone the abdominal, buttock and leg muscles, as well as greatly improving pelvic health and flexibility.

Dancing is healthy, therapeutic and enjoyable because it promotes flexibility in both body and mind – to dance well we need let go and allow our energy to flow.

Arm stretches
tiryaka tadasana

❶ Stand with your feet slightly apart, arms at your sides. ❷ Stretch your arms out in front of you. Link your fingers, palms facing in. Breathe in. ❸ Turn your palms out. Breathe out. ❹ Breathe in and raise your arms slowly above your head. Stretch upward with your arms straight and your palms facing the ceiling. ❺ Stretch to the right, extending the left side of your body. Breathe out. ❻ Breathe in and return to center. ❼ Stretch to the left, extending the right side of your body. Breathe out. Breathe in and return to center. ❽ Breathe out and lower your arms to your sides. ❾ Stand in the start position for a few moments then repeat the sequence twice more.

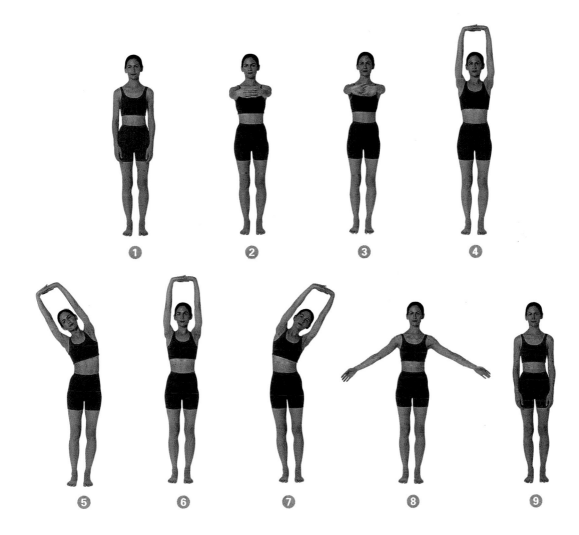

Stretching upward energizes the body, especially when accompanied by yogic breathing. Side stretches keep joints flexible and open the vertebrae laterally. In everyday life the spine is not usually extended in this way.

The movements of these arm stretches signify an ability to move the upper part of our body with the winds of change yet to keep our feet firmly planted on the ground.

Forward bend
utthanasana

1 Stand with your feet slightly apart and your hands together in the prayer position. **2** Breathing in, raise both hands above your head, palms facing. Keep your arms straight and parallel, your fingers pointing up. **3** Breathing out, fold your arms above your head. Grip your elbows. Breathe in. **4** Breathing out, bend at your hips and knees as if going to sit down. **5** Bend forward and lower your palms to the floor. **6** Breathing in, let your fingers slide over your feet, ankles and the fronts of your legs. Straighten your knees and slowly stand up. **7** Breathing out, bring your hands back to the prayer position. Repeat the sequence, reversing the clasp of your elbows.

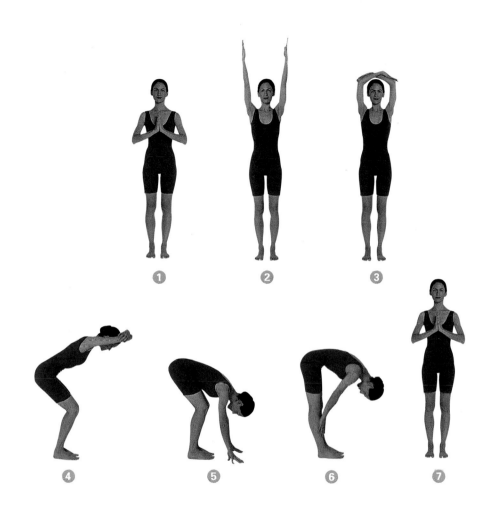

This *asana* sequence makes you feel refreshed and invigorated, and regular practice builds your energy levels so that you don't tire so easily. You should approach this sequence slowly. If you have any lower-back problems or suffer from high blood pressure, consult your doctor or a qualified yoga therapist first.

This sequence tones your back muscles and helps to make your spine more flexible.

The cat
marjari-asana

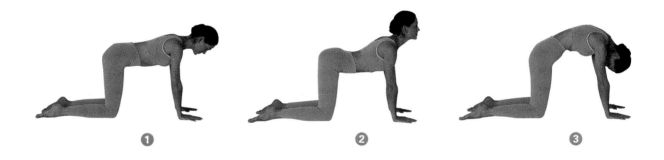

① ② ③

This posture frees the spine and neck, improves the circulation, and stimulates the digestive tract and spinal fluids. It is a useful posture for women who experience menstrual cramps. The Cat posture also teaches you to coordinate your breath with your movements.

When you practice this posture, focus on the eyebrow chakra (ajna) **as you breathe in and on the sacral chakra** (swadhistana) **as you breathe out.**

1 Start on your hands and knees. Your hands should be directly under your shoulders with your fingers spread out and your middle fingers pointing forward. Your knees should be directly under your hips, with your thighs at right angles to your calves. **2** As you breathe in, slowly roll your eyes upward and then raise your head, neck and shoulders to follow. Allow your spine to dip and your hips to tilt so that your tailbone points upward. **3** As you breathe out, pull your abdominal muscles up toward your spine and allow your hips to tilt forward and your head to come down so that your spine curves upward. Repeat this sequence up to 5 times.

Downward-facing dog
adho mukha shvanasana

1 Start on your hands and knees. Your palms should be shoulders' width apart and your fingers should be spread with your middle fingers pointing forward. Take a moment or two to breathe in and out, then curl your toes under your feet. **2** Breathing in, let your knees come off the floor – imagine that you are being pulled up into the air by the base of your spine. Keep your knees bent and allow your chest to come close to your thighs. **3** Breathing out, try to release your heels so that they sink to the floor. Straighten your knees and lift your hips. Relax your neck and shoulders. Keep breathing. Hold the posture for as long as you feel comfortable and steady.

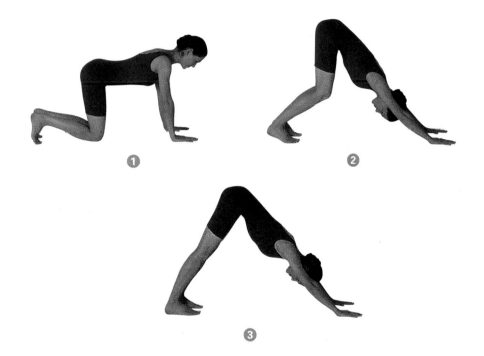

Downward-facing dog strengthens your arm and leg muscles, your spine and the long bones of your arms and legs. It also stimulates the circulation and nerves in the upper back and shoulders. When you practice this posture, focus your attention on the throat chakra (*vishuddhi*).

Yoga teacher Swami Ajnananda always used to remind his students that the Downward-facing dog is a posture in which they could meditate!

Pose of the child
supta shashankasana

1 Start on your hands and knees. **2** Push back, sit on your heels and extend your arms. Gently rest your forehead on the floor. Feel the stretch and allow your spine to lengthen. Sink more deeply into the posture with each out-breath. **3** Make your hands into fists. Slide them back, resting one on top of the other under your forehead. **4** Sit back on your heels with your palms on your knees. **5** Breathing in, raise your arms in an arc in front of your body, above your head. Keep your palms facing in and your elbows straight. Breathe out and lower your arms. **6** Gently lower your forehead to the floor and extend your arms behind you, resting them by your sides.

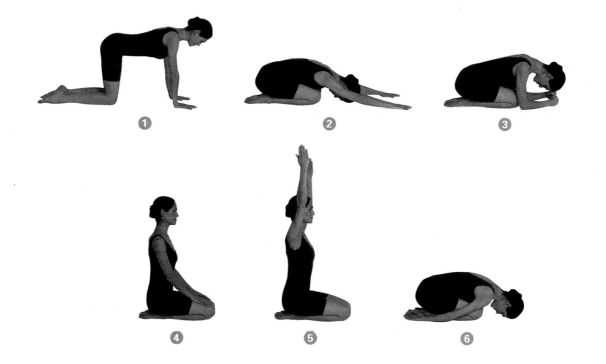

This series relaxes the spinal ligaments and stretches the back muscles. The final posture relieves compression on the intervertebral disks which become compacted when standing. It is a wonderfully relaxing posture.

If you find it difficult to sit back on your heels, try putting a cushion under your buttocks and sit on this. You can even try one under your feet as well.

Leg lift
ardha shalabhasana

1 Lie face down and fold your arms in front of you, with one forearm on top of the other. Turn your head to one side and rest it on your arms. Focus on your breath – let it flow naturally. **2** Move your arms to your sides, palms facing upward. Your forehead should rest on the floor. **3** Breathe in and raise your left leg from the hip. Keep the knee straight. Breathe out and gently lower your leg. Repeat up to 5 times. **4** Repeat Step 3 with your right leg. **5** Press down with your arms and raise both legs together. Repeat up to 5 times. Return to Step 1 and rest with your head facing in the opposite direction.

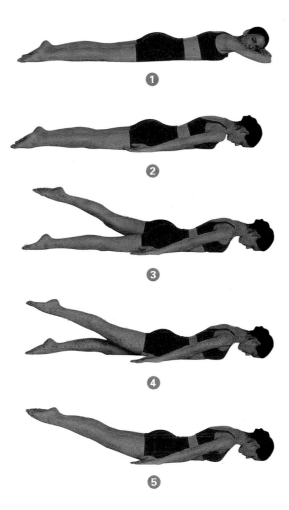

The Leg lift is helpful for beginners as it stimulates the nerves in the lower back and helps to strengthen the back muscles. Synchronizing breath and movement helps to develop concentration. When you practice the Leg lift, focus your attention on the sacral chakra (*swadhisthana*).

Don't attempt to lift both legs together until you are entirely comfortable raising the legs individually.

The cobra
bhujangasana

1 Lie flat on your stomach with your legs extended and your feet together. Fold your arms and rest your head on them. Relax your leg muscles. **2** Bring your hands underneath and slightly to the sides of your shoulders, with your fingers pointing forward. Keep your elbows close to the sides of your body and rest your forehead on the floor. Relax your whole body, particularly your lower back. **3** As you breathe in, slowly raise your head, neck and shoulders off the floor (your hips should remain firmly on the floor). Breathe out and slowly lower your body back to the starting position with your head facing in the other direction. Repeat this sequence up to 5 times.

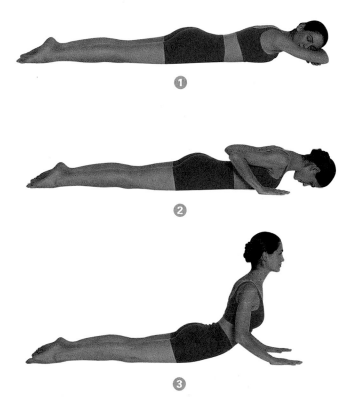

The Cobra strengthens the abdominal and back muscles and is beneficial for lower-back problems. It can also ease gynecological problems and, because it works on the abdominal organs, it aids digestion. It is a wonderful posture for activating energy from the base chakra (*muladhara*) to the third-eye chakra (*ajna*).

People with ulcers, hernias or intestinal problems should not practice this asana without expert guidance.

The thunderbolt
vajrasana

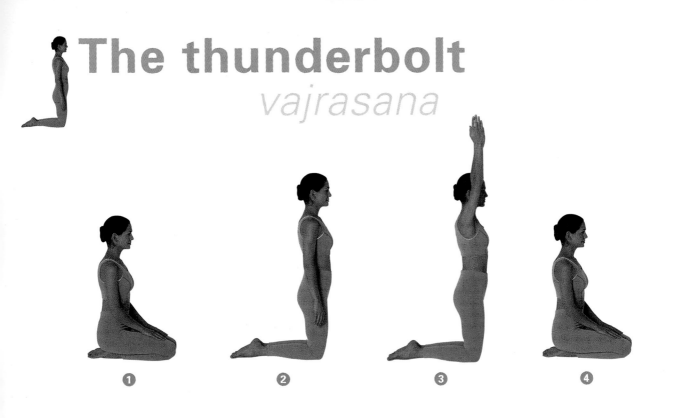

① ② ③ ④

Sitting back on your heels is a wonderful meditation posture for people who cannot sit cross-legged (even those with sciatica) and it activates life-force energy, or *prana*.

If you have varicose veins or poor circulation in the legs, place a cushion between your heels and buttocks to relieve pressure when you sit back on your heels. You may also find it helpful to put a cushion between the floor and your feet.

❶ Sit back on your heels. Your insteps should be on the floor and your big toes should be touching, with the inside edges of your feet close together. Rest your hands palms down on your knees. Make sure that your spine is straight. **❷** As you breathe in, come up from sitting into a kneeling position. Now breathe out. **❸** As you breathe in, raise your arms in an arc in front of you, bringing your hands above your head, palms facing each other. Lower your arms in an arc as you breathe out. **❹** Breathe in. Sit back on your heels as you breathe out. Repeat this sequence up to 5 times.

The butterfly
poorna titali

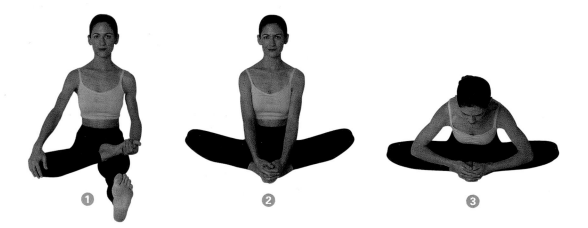

This is a good preparation for the Lotus posture and for sitting in meditation. The Butterfly posture relieves inner-thigh tension and is helpful if you sit or stand for long periods.

It is said that the effect created by the movement of a butterfly's wings in one part of the world can trigger a tornado thousands of miles away. So be gentle in your practice!

1 Sit on the floor with your left leg extended. Rest your right foot on your left thigh, holding your toes with your left hand. Gently clasp your right knee with your right hand. Breathe in and out, raising and lowering your knee several times. Change legs and repeat. **2** Bend both knees and bring the soles of the feet together. Clasp your toes. Slide your heels toward your body. Straighten your spine and breathe in. Breathe out and lower your knees to the floor. Concentrate on counting your breaths and relaxing into the posture. **3** Bend your elbows and, working from the lower back, lower your body so that your chest comes toward the floor. Breathe in. Sit upright.

Easy spinal twist
sukhasana matsyendrasana

1 Sit with your legs crossed at the ankles, your back straight and your palms on your knees. **2** Breathing in deeply, raise your arms out to the sides. **3** Rest your right palm on your left knee. Breathe out. Turn your left palm to face backward. **4** Swing your left arm behind you and rest your palm or fingertips on the floor. Use this arm to help keep your spine straight and upright. **5** Breathing out, gradually turn your body to the left, feeling energy moving up the spine as you do so. Look over your left shoulder. Breathe in and out. Slowly release the posture as you breathe out. Return to Step 1 and repeat the sequence, twisting to the right.

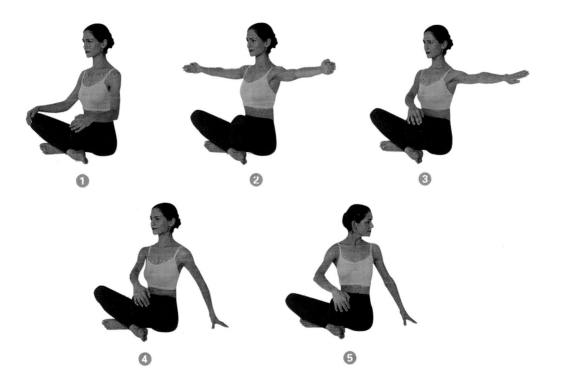

Twisting postures give the spine a wonderful workout, releasing enormous amounts of tension and flooding the spinal nerves with nutrients and energy. They open the heart chakra (*anahata*) and help to bring a greater volume of air into the lungs. They have a strong influence on the abdominal muscles as they stretch and compress them.

If you find it difficult to sit cross-legged on the floor, you can sit on a folded blanket or a firm cushion. Be careful not to over-extend yourself and twist more than your natural flexibility will permit.

The half-moon
ardha chandrasana

1 Stand with your feet slightly apart, breathe in and raise your arms above your head. Clasp your elbows. **2** Breathe out and bend forward at your waist, bending your knees if necessary. **3** Place your hands on the floor. Step your right foot back, keeping your heel off the floor. **4** Lower your right knee to the floor and straighten your toes. Breathe out. **5** Swing your arms forward and above your head. Keep your elbows straight and palms facing. Breathe in. Sink into your hips. Focus on your breathing. **6** Lower your palms to the floor and straighten both legs. Breathe out. **7** Swing your right foot forward and stand up. Repeat on the other side.

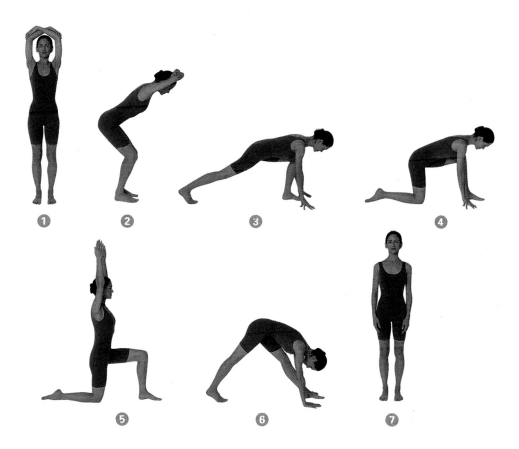

The Half-moon posture opens out the front of the chest and stretches the lungs. It strengthens the entire skeletal structure and, because it works strongly on the chest and neck, it frequently relieves respiratory ailments, including sore throats, coughs and colds. All in all it is a very invigorating posture!

When you practice this posture, focus on the sacral chakra (swadhisthana) **and on controlled movement and balance.**

The archer
akarana dhanurasana

1 Stand with your feet hips' width apart. **2** Step your left foot forward by a leg length and turn in your right foot so the instep aligns with your left heel. **3** Turn your hips and upper body to the right. Raise your arms sidewise to shoulder height. **4** Look along both arms – check that they are level with your shoulders. Extend your fingers. **5** Fold your right arm in toward your chest with your elbow at shoulder height, as if holding the string of a bow. Look along your left arm. Breathe in and out in the posture for as long as you can remain steady. Repeat on the other side.

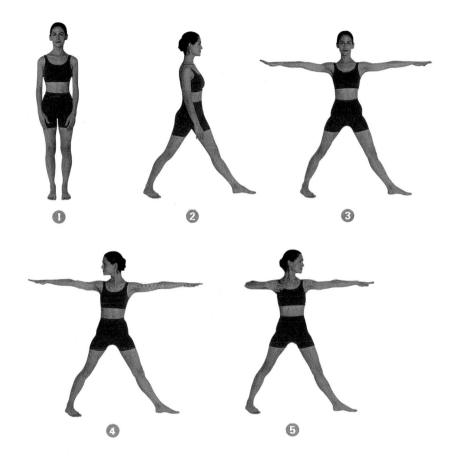

This posture works on the short, deep muscles in the neck and shoulders, and is excellent for releasing tension. To enhance tension release, try sliding the bent arm forward as you breathe out and bring it back as you breathe in.

Lord Krishna advised the warrior Arjuna to learn the wisdom of skill in action: "By this I mean perfect balance, unshakeable equanimity, poise and peace of mind." *Bhagavad Gita* (2:50)

The triangle
trikonasana

1 Stand with your feet wide apart. Breathe in. Raise and stretch your arms out to the side. **2** Turn your left leg out 90 degrees and push your right heel slightly out to the right. Breathe out. **3** Breathe in. Stretch your left hand down to hold your left ankle and your right hand straight up. **4** Breathe out. Bring your right hand down past your right ear and stretch it out to the left. Breathe in. Stand up, arms outstretched. **5** Lower your arms, and point your feet forward. Repeat on the other side.

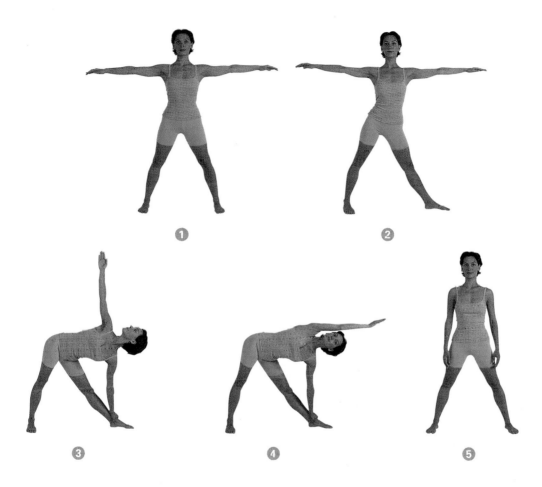

This yoga pose opens up the hip and shoulder girdles to allow the free movement of energy, and helps to trim the waist, making it more supple.

For maximum benefit take your time and do this exercise slowly – it creates a really satisfying stretch.

The bridge
kandharasana

1 Lie flat on your back with your arms near your sides and your palms facing down. Tilt your head slightly so that your chin moves toward your throat and the back of your neck lengthens. **2** Bend your knees and put the soles of your feet flat on the floor (first the left foot and then the right). Your feet and knees should be hips' width apart and your feet should be parallel. **3** Press down on your palms and, as you breathe in, raise your hips off the floor. Hold the posture. Breathe. Raise your hips a little more on each in-breath. **4** Breathe out and lower your hips. Stretch out your legs and then return to rest in the starting position. Repeat up to 5 times.

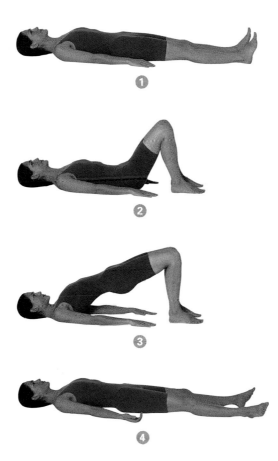

This posture massages the abdominal and female reproductive organs, improving digestion and easing menstrual problems. It can also help to realign the spine and relieve backache. People with ulcers or hernias and women in late pregnancy should avoid this posture or seek expert guidance.

When you practice this posture, focus on the heart chakra (anahata) **or the throat chakra** (vishuddhi).

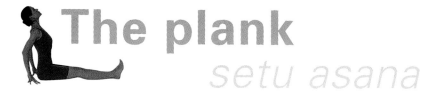

The plank
setu asana

1 Sit on the floor with your legs extended, your spine straight and your hands at your sides just behind your hips. **2** Breathe in and lift your chest, gently arching your back. Breathing out, sit upright. **3** Take your hands a little further behind you so that your upper body is at about 45 degrees to the floor. Keep your arms straight. **4** Breathe in, roll your shoulders back and allow your chest to rise and your hips to lift off the floor. Gently point your toes, relax your neck and look up. Breathe. Try to raise your hips a little more on each in-breath. **5** Breathe out and lower your hips. **6** Gently lie down with your legs bent and your arms away from your sides. Relax.

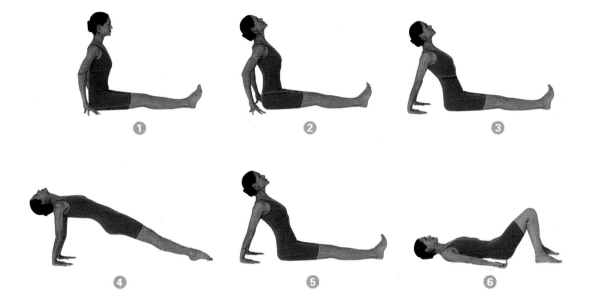

The Plank strengthens the arms, legs and the lumbar region of the spine. It is a good counterpose to forward-bending postures. You should avoid it, however, if you have high blood pressure, heart problems or a stomach ulcer. Focus on the solar-plexus chakra (*manipura*) during your practice.

When you can hold this posture comfortably, try lifting your pelvic area higher into the air. You can also try it with your hands facing backward and even lifting one arm or leg off the ground. Have fun!

Half-shoulder stand
vipareeta karani

1 Lie on your back, arms at your sides, palms facing down. **2** Slide your feet toward your buttocks with your soles flat on the floor. **3** Push down with your hands and use your abdominal muscles to raise your knees. **4** Raise your legs and hips. Support your lower back with your hands. Your legs should be at a 45 degree angle to the floor, your feet relaxed and your elbows close together. Hold the posture and breathe. **5** Bring your knees to your chest, put your hands on the floor for support and slowly roll out of the pose, one vertebra at a time. **6** Lie down with your feet apart and your arms by your sides, palms facing up. Relax your body and breathe.

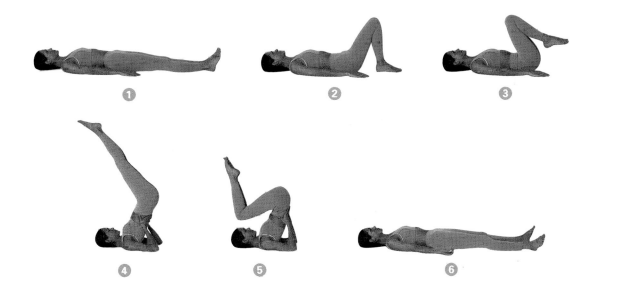

This posture stimulates the thyroid gland, relieves headaches and helps to calm mental and emotional disturbance. Do not practice it if you suffer from high blood pressure, weak blood vessels in the eyes or heart complaints. It should also be avoided during menstruation and the final stages of pregnancy.

"One achieves serenity by focusing on the inner light." *Yoga Sutras of Patanjali* (1:36)

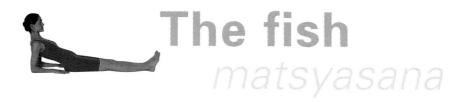

The fish
matsyasana

1 Sit on the floor, legs extended, spine upright and hands behind your hips. **2** Breathing out, lower yourself to the floor using your forearms for support. **3** Slide your hands toward your feet. Raise your chest and rest the back of your head on the floor. Keep your chest raised as high as possible. Breathe in and out for as long as you are comfortable. **4** To release, slide your hands under your lower back, press down on your hands and elbows and lift your head. **5** Lie down. Release your hands, link your fingers and cradle your head in your hands. Pull your knees toward your chest. Cross your ankles and let your knees drop. Relax totally and focus on your breath.

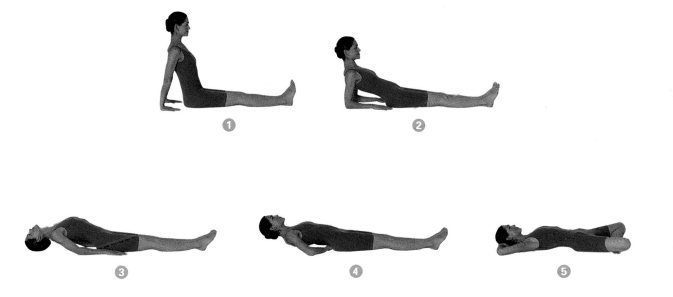

This posture opens up the chest and neck and is useful for abdominal and respiratory complaints, including colds and 'flu. It is also a very energizing posture. Take care getting in and out of this posture and avoid it altogether if you are pregnant, or suffer from heart disease or other serious health problems.

When you practice this posture, focus on the heart chakra (anahata) **in Step 3 and on the solar-plexus chakra** (manipura) **for the final relaxation.**

Our energy levels are linked to the cycle of the Sun
– we naturally have more energy during daylight.

Kinesiology is particularly good at the start of the
day – it improves coordination, vision and hearing.

Qigong exercises are great at any time to
provide a rapid, quick-fix boost of energy.

chapter seven

Energize your day

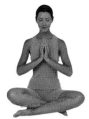

Understanding the ebb and flow of our energy levels through the day is important for living life to the full.

We all have different body clocks: some people feel sluggish and find it hard to function first thing in the morning; many have a dip in energy after lunch; and most of us feel drained at the end of a busy day. By learning to recognize and anticipate the fluctuations in our energy levels we can take steps to replenish our reserves to meet particular challenges at different times in our schedule. In this chapter there are exercises to improve our energy levels when we rise, after lunch and in the evening, as well as others that can quickly boost our energy flow whenever we need vitality most.

The five-finger fix

1 Rest the tips of the thumb and four fingers of your left hand over your navel. Place the thumb and index finger of your right hand just below your collarbones. Wiggle all your fingers for 10 seconds to energize the meridians. **2** Keeping your left hand over your navel, place your right index finger on the middle of your top lip and your thumb on the middle of your lower lip, and rub these points for 10 seconds. **3** Place your right hand flat on the base of your spine and massage this spot for 10 seconds while still keeping your left hand over your navel. Repeat with your right hand over your navel and your left hand in the three positions.

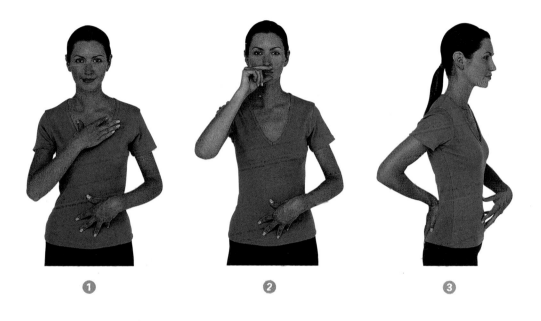

1 2 3

Massaging the two points below the collarbones helps to balance the energy flow in the kidney meridian. The fingers placed around the navel stimulate the flow of all the meridians in the navel area. The index finger and thumb placed on the lips connect the two energy reservoirs – the Governor and Conception vessels. The different actions of the two hands, and the points they massage, encourage the flow of electrical energy through the brain.

If you wake up feeling "out of sorts", kinesiology will point your energy back in the right direction.

Morning stretch

1 Stand up straight with your hands in the prayer position. **2** Breathing in, raise your arms in an arc above your head, fold your arms and clasp your elbows. Breathing out, bend forward at the hips. Extend your spine. **3** Lower your hands to the floor. **4** Step your feet back (right then left). Lift your hips up high and drop your heels to the floor. **5** Breathe out and bring your knees to the floor. Breathe in, raise your head, tilt your hips and let your spine hollow. **6** Breathe out, lift your abdomen, lower your head and look between your legs. Repeat Steps 5 and 6 twice. **7** Push back, sit on your heels and stretch from your fingertips to the base of your spine. **8** Sit upright. Put your palms on your knees. Focus on your breathing.

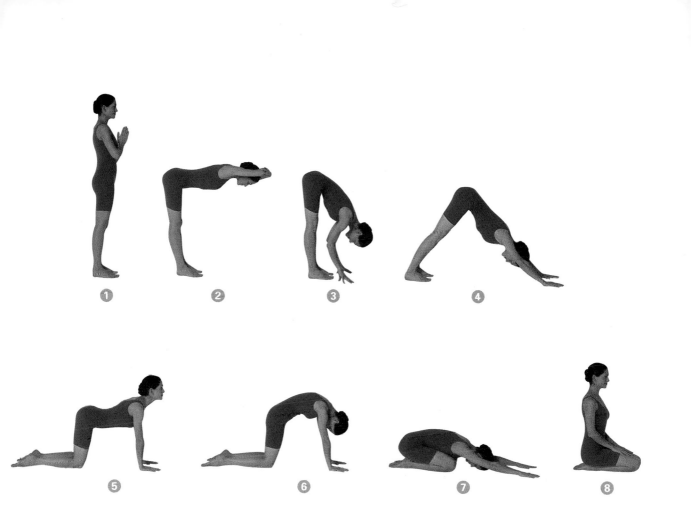

Give yourself at least 10 or 15 minutes for this sequence – it will invigorate you, balance your energy and prepare you for the day.

In the final stage of this sequence, close your eyes and make a resolution for the day. Open your eyes and smile.

The cross crawl

1 Lift one knee and swing the opposite arm so that the elbow touches the knee. **2** Lift the other knee and opposite arm in the same way. Looking at a plain wall, march like this 10 times, on the spot. Continue for another 10 marches, this time rolling your eyes widely in a clockwise movement. Repeat the sequence, this time rolling your eyes counter-clockwise. Now march another 10 times, moving your eyes in a large figure of eight. **3** Raise your right arm and right leg simultaneously 10 times, while following the above sequence of eye movements. Now raise your left arm and left leg, and march 10 times, repeating the eye movements once more. Finish by repeating Steps 1 and 2.

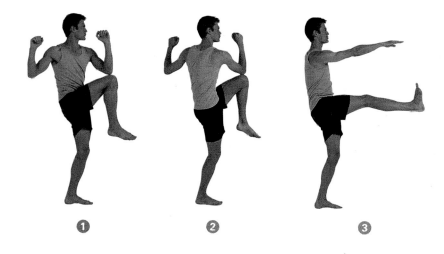

① ② ③

Kinesiology exercises are specifically designed to exercise the brain as well as the body. They improve the connections between the right and left hemispheres of the brain by coordinating movements between the two halves of the body. They are beneficial for everyone, but particularly for people with learning difficulties and dyslexia.

This exercise is based on, and named after, the crawling movements of babies.

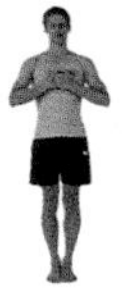

Brain coordination

1 Stand, feet together, eyes closed, with your arms at shoulder height out to the sides, palms forward. **2** Slowly bring your arms together until your palms meet – keep trying if this does not happen first time – it's more difficult than you might think. Link your fingers and imagine that you are joining the two sides of your brain. **3** Bring your hands in to your chest as if you are drawing in your whole self. Rest with one hand on top of the other. **4** Relax, hands by your sides, eyes closed, and enjoy the calm, satisfied feeling of your brain being in balance.

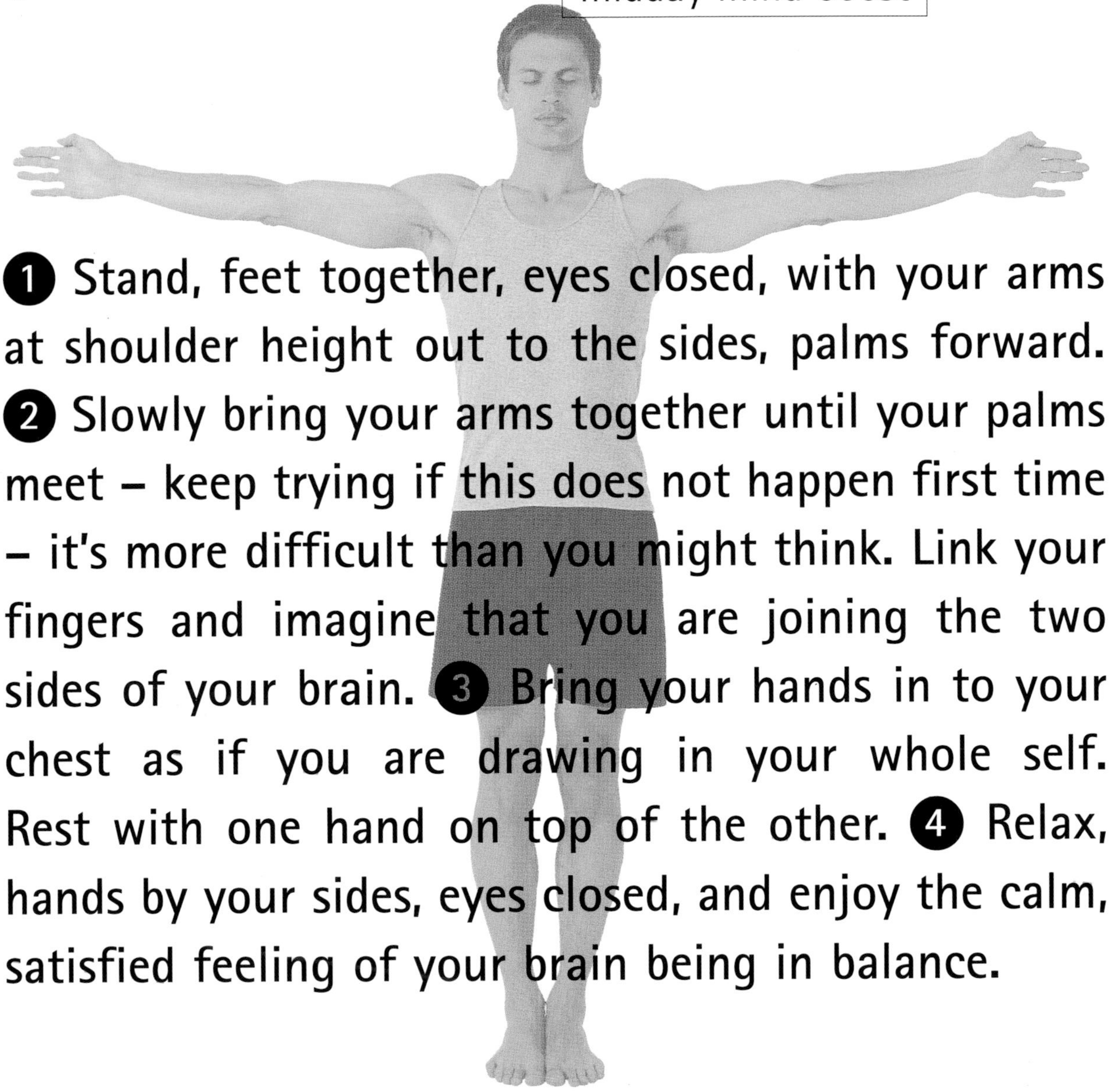

ENERGIZE YOUR DAY

230

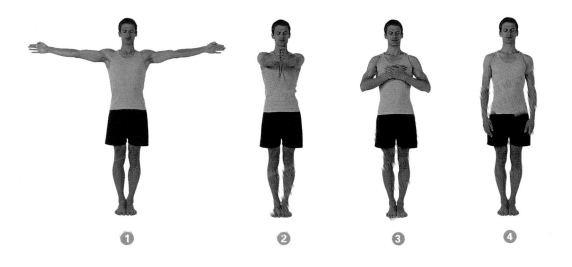

This kinesiology exercise simultaneously stimulates both hemispheres of the brain so that you think and move in a more coordinated way. It also helps to calm and balance the emotions by integrating confused and conflicting thoughts.

Try this in your lunch hour – ask your colleagues to join in too.

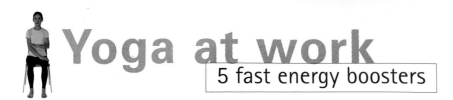

Yoga at work

5 fast energy boosters

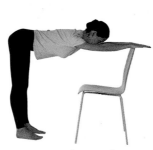

Forward extension

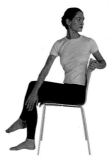

Spinal twist

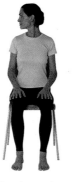

Head rotation

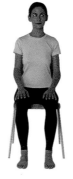

Eye relaxation

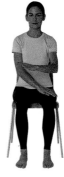

Knee taps

When you start to run out of energy at work or at home during the day, these simple yoga practices can be invaluable.

These postures are even more effective if you concentrate on your breath and allow your mind to clear.

Forward extension Stand facing a chair. Bend and hold the back of the chair so that your legs are at 90 degrees to your body. Elongate your spine. Stretch your fingers.

Spinal twist Sit upright and cross your left leg over your right. Put your right hand over your left knee, your left hand on the chair back. Lift up your spine and twist your body to the left. Repeat on the other side.

Head rotation Sit or stand. Breathing out, turn your head to the right. Breathing in, return to center. Breathing out, turn to the left. Do this for 2 minutes.

Eye relaxation Imagine a clockface around your eyes. Look at 12 o'clock and count each numeral clockwise. Now do this counterclockwise. Repeat several times.

Knee taps Cross your arms and simply tap each knee in turn. Try to synchronize your breathing with the taps.

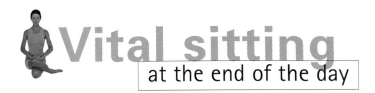

Vital sitting
at the end of the day

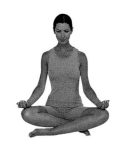

The meditation

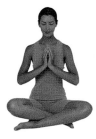

The prayer

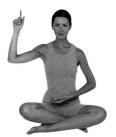

The energy conduit

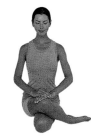

The energy harmonizer

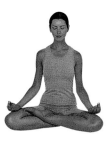

The half lotus

The above qigong and yoga sitting postures open out the hip and shoulder girdles, increasing energy flow up the spine. Spend 5 minutes practicing one of them at the end of the day – close your eyes, breathe deeply and relax.

In sitting postures, when the hands are in an open position they receive energy; when they are held close to the body they conduct energy inward.

The meditation Sit cross-legged, keeping your spine straight (but not strained) and rest the backs of your hands on your knees.

The prayer Touch the tips of your fingers and the heels of your hands together in a prayer position to energize and nourish the heart chakra (*anahata*).

The energy conduit Point one index finger skyward to draw down *qi*, your wrist facing forward. Cup your other palm horizontally in front of your navel.

The energy harmonizer Sit on one heel with your upper leg crossed as far as possible over the lower leg, your hands on top of each other on your knee.

The half lotus Sit cross-legged and bring one foot up onto the opposite calf. Place your hands on your knees, keeping the palms open.

Evening practice

Here are some simple meditative practices. Take time in the evening to relax and let go of the day's events. Try to practice with "conscious awareness": observe your thoughts but do not allow them to take over. Instead of judging your performance, simply think: "Now I am practicing yoga." Start by sitting comfortably with your back straight.

Humming-bee practice Close your eyes and relax. Close the flaps of your ears with your index fingers. Imagine a humming bee inside your head. Breathe in. Breathe out and make the even, controlled noise of a humming bee. Repeat up to 5 times. This produces a meditational state and eases stress and insomnia.

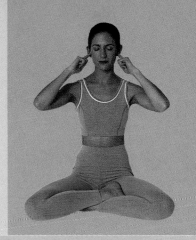

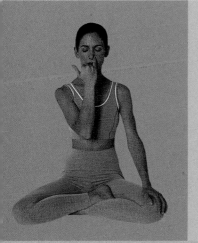

Alternate-nostril breathing Hold the right nostril closed with the thumb and breathe into the left nostril. Close the left nostril with the little finger, release the right nostril and breathe out. Breathe in through the right nostril, then close it with your thumb. Release your left nostril and breathe out. Repeat several times.

Visualization of chakras and colors Imagine drawing up red-colored energy from the earth into your base chakra. Visualize the color changes (red, orange, yellow, green, blue and violet) as the energy ascends the differently colored chakras. At the crown chakra the energy becomes white, creating an envelope around you.

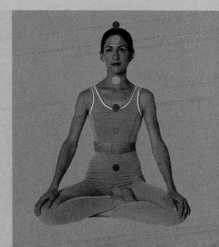

Bedtime relaxation

This is a very powerful relaxation practice that allows you to let go of physical discomfort and emotional blockages, as well as improve your memory and concentration. The candle-gazing practice helps to balance your nervous system, relieving stress and insomnia, and enhancing sleep.

"The person who is able to control the mind and engage in actions without attachment is able to excel." *Bhagavad Gita* (3:7)

Light a candle and your favorite incense. Spend a few minutes thinking over the events of the day and then let go of these thoughts. Make an agreement with yourself that for the next 15–20 minutes your thoughts will be on the practice of relaxation and meditation. Sit in a comfortable position with your back straight. Spend some minutes looking at the candle flame. Close your eyes and hold the image in your mind. When the image disappears, open your eyes and look at the flame again. Repeat this a few times.

Remain sitting or lie down on the floor in the relaxation pose, *shavasana* (see pp.166–7), but do not fall asleep. Practice yoga breathing (see pp.172–3) or alternate-nostril breathing (see p.237) for a few minutes and then scan your body, looking for tension. Breathe into any areas of tension and, when you breathe out, allow them to soften and release.

Now visualize the candle flame on the screen of your mind. Allow it to be small at first but, as you watch, see it grow bigger and brighter, washing over your body, bringing peace, love and compassion. Allow the flame to fill every aspect of your interior space and then let it focus at the heart chakra (*anahata*).

Allow this image to fade and bring your awareness to the breath at the tip of your nose. Then gradually become aware of your body, starting with your fingers and toes. When you are ready, gently open your eyes.

Sensing the energy

1 Stand, feet shoulders' width apart, knees slightly bent, arms by your sides. **2** Bring your hands in front of your abdomen, palms facing inward. Spend 2 minutes visualizing a ball of energy emanating from your abdomen, filling your hands. **3** Slowly, move your hands apart and imagine the ball of energy growing between them. Keep this position for 1 minute. **4** Now visualize the ball of energy contracting, as it pulls your hands in toward each other. Repeat several times until you can feel the energy expand and contract. **5** Draw your hands in toward your abdomen and imagine the ball of energy contracting back inside into a small spark. Wiggle your hands and shake your fingers.

ENERGIZE YOUR DAY

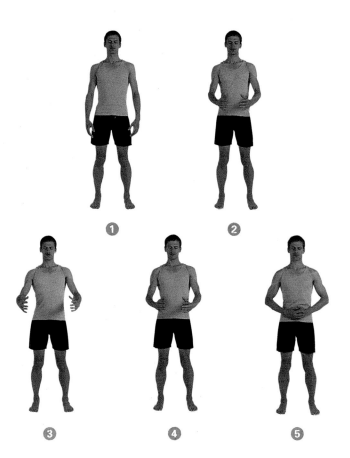

This qigong exercise can give you an energy boost at any time of the day. It helps to increase the flow in the energy center known as the lower dantien, which is located deep in the abdomen. According to Chinese tradition, the lower dantien is the seat of our being and the source of our vitality.

You will know when you succeed in feeling the energy between your hands – they will tingle or warm up.

Energy first-aid

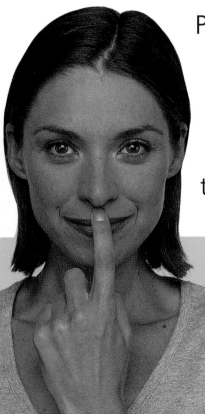

Pressing the acupoints encourages the body to maintain its natural energy equilibrium and regulates the energy flow. The following acupressure exercises provide quick-fix self-help to restore the balance in your body.

Governor Vessel 26 Located a third of the way down the groove in the middle of the upper lip. To make you more alert, or to relieve feelings of faintness, press this point 3 times with your index finger, for 7–10 seconds each.

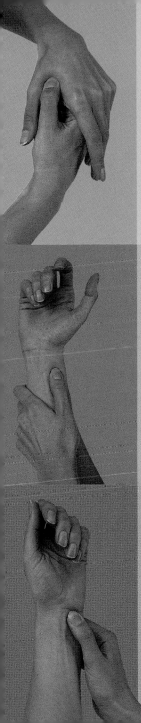

Large Intestine 4 Found in the fleshy web between the thumb and the index finger. Stimulating the energy flow in this meridian helps to treat diarrhea, rashes and toothache. Press this acupoint 3 times, on both hands, for 10–15 seconds each. It is not advisable to press this point on a pregnant woman.

Lung 7 Located on the forearm, $1^{1}/_{2}$ in below the wrist fold, on the same side as the thumb, in the hollow behind the wrist bone. Pressing this acupoint helps to increase the energy flow to the lungs to combat respiratory problems, common colds and headaches. Press hard with your thumb 3 times, on both wrists, for 7–10 seconds each.

Heart 7 Found down below the little finger, on the inside of the wrist, just behind the wrist crease. Stimulating this acupoint helps to counteract irritability and to treat insomnia. Support your wrist with the fingers of your other hand, then press this point 3 times, on both wrists, for 7–10 seconds each.

Index

Acknowledgments

The Publishers would like to thank:

Models: Helen Brumby, Tim Cummins, Tara Fraser, Caroline Long, Kerry Norton

Make–up artists/hairdressers: Elizabeth Lawson, Evelynne Stoikou

Authors Nic Rowley and Kirsten Hartvig would like to thank the following people for their help and inspiration:

Jill Byrne, Geoffrey Cannon, Judy Dean, Peter Firebrace, Lilly Jensen, Allan Hartvig, Tessa Hodsdon, Jennifer Maughan, Anna Mews, Kathy Mitchison, Susie Mitchison, Françoise Nassivet, Liz Pearson, François Salies, Katinka Thielemans, Joyce Thomas, Linda Wilkinson, Ric Wilkinson, Jackie Young

Nic Rowley's and Kirsten Hartvig's website is at www.labergerie.net